Best Home Remedies For Acne

Your Total Guide To Natural Acne Treatments & The Best Natural Acne Treatment Recipes

I0426551

ISBN: 13: 978-1494245092

The advice contained in this material might not be suitable for everyone. The author believes that a natural and holistic approach to health and maintaining the body's natural balance. This material is written for the express purpose of sharing educational information and scientific research gathered from the studies and experiences of the author, healthcare professionals, scientists, nutritionists and informed health advocates.

The author recognizes that within scientific and medical fields there are widely divergent viewpoints and opinions and therefore it is the readers responsibility to investigate all aspects of any decision before committing him or herself to any treatment. The author obtained the information from sources she believes to be reliable, but she neither implies nor intends any guarantee of accuracy for specific cases or individuals.

Before beginning any practice relating to health, diet or exercise, it is recommended that you first obtain the consent and advice of a licensed health care professional. The contents of this e-book are not a replacement for professional advice. Always consult your own Doctor or medical professional before starting any treatment, process or action.

The author assumes no responsibility for the choices you make after your review of the information contained herein and your consultation with a licensed healthcare professional. The author, publisher and distributors particularly disclaim any liability, loss, or risk taken by individuals who directly or indirectly act on the information contained in this e-book. The author believes the advice presented here is sound, but readers cannot hold the author, publisher and distributors responsible for either the actions they take or the results of those actions.

Please note that although the oils, recipes and remedies presented in this book are known to be the most gentle to sensitive skins and scalps: as with any natural substance some oils such as thyme can in some individuals cause mild irritation on rare occasions and some oils should

NOT be used at all while pregnant. It is recommended that as a precaution you should patch test all oils/formulas before application to skin.

CONTENTS

INTRODUCTION

You want to stop hiding behind makeup and concealers and to be proud of the skin you're in – I get it completely!

And moreover you want to stop paying for expensive creams, washes and goop that's made by people who don't understand you or your (unique) skin. You want a natural solution that doesn't employ a "throw a bazooka at it" kind of attitude!

As someone who has suffered from periodic acne and scalp pimples for many years, and having endured watching my son and partner deal with severe acne for years, I know the pain, frustration and annoyance it brings.

As a natural body and skin therapist I have also dealt with (and happy to say, dealt to) all sorts of skin and scalp conditions (I used to suffer from severe scalp pimples and itching myself too). I have spent years of testing, research, trial and error I have discovered many successful treatments for acne among many other skin conditions. I know from hard earned experience what works and what doesn't. I also acknowledge that everyone is different, no ones skin is the same, we are all made up of different combinations of genes, we come from different environments, and so we need to deal with acne with these factors in mind.

I am not purporting this to be a miracle one treatment cures all answer, (there is no such thing) but - over time hopefully a very short time, your acne will be a thing of the past. Your skin will heal, and (usually over 7 to 15 days) you will start to see a significant improvement that only gets better and better as you use the right products you made yourself at home.

You won't find me recommending expensive creams prescriptions or nasty chemicals…just all natural solutions that work LONG TERM.

I'm going to give you some diet tips, tried tested recipes, and long term beauty ideas for gorgeous skin.

There are also the longer term aspects of acne to consider, which include how to deal with acne scars so you can leave behind the legacy of scarred damaged skin and get on with an acne free life.

The absolute truth is, there is no quick fix for acne and blemishes or one specific magic recipe for all skin types to make them go away forever. Acne and oil related pimples will still happen from time to time (I know that stinks, but you can't prevent the odd one poking it's head up every now and then). What you can do however, is change the environment they like to develop in, making your skin an inhospitable place for acne bacteria to grow.

I'm going to share with you a whole bunch of skincare tips and recipes to try. Most will work, a few won't depending on your body and skin type. (If you are allergic to any of the foods I suggest in these recipes, DO NOT try using them on your skin!).

Remember your acne and oily skin may not disappear overnight, you will need to change a few things about how you care for your skin. But...

By incorporating a few good dietary habits (no I'm not suggesting you become a vegan or eat only lettuce), and good skin routines using ALL NATURAL skin care ingredients and recipes you can make at home, you CAN get clear blemish free skin.

WHAT ACTUALLY IS ACNE?

Acne is a dermatological term that describes clogged and infected pores/hair follicles, red lumps, pimples and lumps or cysts that can occur on the face, neck, chest, back, shoulders, and upper arms. Acne can be a painful and embarrassing experience for those who live with it.

Although acne is a more common occurrence in teenagers, it is not limited to this age group. Acne can even be problematic for people in their forties. For some people, acne only lasts for a few years through puberty and their early twenties. But for others, it can be a reoccurring problem for decades. Whatever the case, the bacteria that causes acne and the physical and emotional discomfort associated with it can be treated.

Acne presents itself (rears its ugly head so to speak) in five ways: comedones (blackheads or whiteheads), papules, pustules, nodules and cysts. Nodules and cysts are much more severe than blackheads or whiteheads.

More severe cases of acne can leave you with potentially permanent scarring in affected areas if not treated with healing ingredients in these recipes.

There are several things that can cause acne. Your pores excrete oils that can become blocked and create the ideal environment for acne bacteria to grow. Hormones and environmental factors can also effect the susceptibility of your body to acne. For instance, if you have been exposed to bacteria from air or water, or microbial transference from fingers etc., then obviously you are more likely to develop pimples.

Hormone imbalances caused by monthly hormonal fluctuations, puberty, stress (causing toxin buildup), health issues and other conditions can increase oil production and therefore the onset of acne. Bacteria can also feed on any dead skin cells that are not removed regularly.

Diet is another factor that effects your skins sebum production. For example, eating high acid producing foods like sugars, meat and alcohol can increase the likelihood of acne breakouts. Consuming oils like safflower oil help to thin sebum and help your skin pass oil more easily from your pores.

You may be starting to see a pattern here, many acne issues come down to how much oil your body is producing, how well you remove dead skin and dirt, and how well your body is at eliminating all of these elements from your pores.

Different Types Of Acne

Acne Vulgaris is the most common type of acne/pimples. It most often affects adolescents (usually right before your prom, job interview or first date) but may persist and become more severe as one reaches adulthood.

Mild to Moderate Acne Vulgaris is characterized by the following:

Whiteheads

Whiteheads are essentially blocked pores which contain trapped sebum, bacteria, and dead skin cells with a white spot appearing on the surface of the skin. Whiteheads generally have a shorter life span than blackheads.

Comedones, another name for blackheads and whiteheads formed one myth says because of too little cleansing, but in fact it has been proven that they are created by a combination of oil, dust and dead skin cells accumulating within the pore itself.

Blackheads

Blackheads are also the result of blocked pores with the surface area of the sebum in the pore having been exposed to the air causing oxidization. Melanin pigment and keratin proteins in dead skin cells can also oxidize contributing to clogged pores and their dark appearance.

Dirt and other grime can also adhere to the surface of blackheads and they usually take longer to clear than whiteheads. Using a good oil based cleanser ....yes I said "oil" for those of you who are saying "what, oil on my already oily skin?". Don't worry, the RIGHT oils won't leave your skin feeling greasy and will help loosen the oils in your blocked pores.

Comedones, the less commonly known term for blackheads, is one of the most common causes of acne, particularly for those who have oily skin. Excess oils accumulate in the sebaceous glands or hair follicles. A blackhead, or open comedone, is open at the surface of the skin. A whitehead, or closed comedone, develops under the surface of the skin. Both blackheads and whiteheads can contribute to the formation of pimples and acne breakouts.

Papules

Papules are red inflamed, red, sore bumps with the absence of a head.

Pustules

A pustule is similar to a whitehead, but is red, tender and inflamed, and may appear as a red circle with a white or yellow "head". (The dreaded zit.)

Severe acne vulgaris may be distinguished by the presence of nodules and cysts.

Nodules / Nodular Acne

Acne nodules are lesions that form hard sore larger lumps (ouch). You should never squeeze (initiate the multi fingered attack on) these lumps as you can spread the infection further into the skin and outward. These lesions can scar and so it is important to let them disappear without aggravating them (don't poke the sleeping bear).

Cysts / Cystic Acne

An acne cyst is similar in appearance to a nodule, but it is pus-filled. The are usually about 1 or 2 inches in diameter and can be very painful. again, squeezing an acne cyst may promote a deeper infection and severe inflammation which extends the life of the lesion.

Severe Acne Types

Many dermatologists and others in the medical field recognize these forms of acne as systemic forms of acne. They can be treated by medical prescription or by including colloidal silver, honey and probiotic yogurt: and even potassium rich bananas as natural "antibiotics" to rebalance skin. If you like yummy smoothies, these are a delicious healthy way of fighting acne from the inside out by balancing bacteria, especially if you add essential fatty acid rich oils to your recipes.

Acne Conglobata

Acne Conglobata is the most severe form of acne vulgaris. This form of extreme acne, generally characterized by the appearance of large and numerous nodules, often interconnected, accompanied by the widespread presence of blackheads. They can become ulcerated, may be very painful and can cause severe scarring. Acne conglobata frequently appears on the back, face, chest, buttocks, upper arms, and tops of your thighs.

It is more common in males and the onset of this acne is typically between 18 and 30 years of age. Acne conglobata can remain in your body for many years dormant until stimulated by dietary, stress or hormonal factors (yes guys it's not just us girls who get hormonal)!

Acne Fulminans

This type of severe acne turns up in what seems like the blink of an eye. It typically picks on young or teenage men. It is very similar in appearance to Acne Conglobata and can leave nasty scarring. What is different and uniques about acne Fulminans is that it also often comes with fever symptoms, aching joints, and can even cause weight loss. This because your body's immune system is having to kick into full gear to deal with it and putting your system under load.

Gram-Negative Folliculitis

Gram-negative folliculitis is a more extreme form of acne caused by a bacterial induced inflammation of the follicles. The condition is characterized by pustules and cysts. Although rare it is caused by a complication of using a specific long-term antibiotic treatment for acne vulgaris.

Why is it called called gram-negative? This relates to the fact that gram is a type of blue stain used in laboratory testing where bacteria organisms that do not stain blue. These nasty little microorganisms are referred to as gram-negative.

Pyoderma Faciale

I'm sorry girls, but this the of severe acne only affects us, usually between the ages of 20 to 40 years. It is characterized by large painful nodules, pustules and sores that can scar. It forms seemingly out of nowhere, and although usually leaves as fast as it arrives, can cause a great deal of damage in a very short time. It usually only stays for 6 months to a year.

Adult Acne

This is a type of acne vulgaris that is usually only present in adults over 30 years of age. If you have never had acne before, thinking you had managed to skip this annoying side effect of puberty, and wondering why you have suddenly developed acne, here are some common causes associated with adult acne:

- Medication (especially epilepsy medications)
- Anabolic steroids (spotty muscle bound bodies)
- Medication or supplements which contain iodine
- Prolonged physical pressure on the skin (straps, harnesses chafing etc)
- Prolonged exposure to chemicals like chlorinated dioxins.
- Metabolic changes and hormonal changes like pregnancy
- Environmental exposure to bacteria (e.g. dairy milking shed, animals, soil etc)
- Reaction or sensitivity to ingredients in skin care or acne products

Acne Rosacea

Rosacea is not actually acne, contrary to the popular myth. Rosacea generally appears as a red lumpy rash around the cheeks, nose, forehead and chin. The redness may be associated with blood vessels close to the surface of the skin. It seems to be more prevalent in women than in men (for whom it tends to be more severe). Rosacea requires a different treatment to acne, so if you have lots of small raised lumps, with red "rosiness" underneath, you may need to try making serums from my website to deal with this specific ailment.

Acne Cosmetica

A form of acne caused by the use of cosmetics - not removing them properly from the skin.

Scalp Acne

Scalp pimples can be caused by a sensitivity or reaction to shampoos especially dandruff shampoos, sulphates and hair dyes.

Excoriated Acne

Acne formed through scrapes and scratches on the skin.

Infantile Acne

This form of acne, known sometimes as milia occurs in newborns and is caused by hormonal changes that have occurred while the fetus was developing in the womb and is generally concentrated on the nose and cheeks. This condition usually clears up in matter of weeks without treatment.

ACNE MYTHS

There are many myths associated with acne conditions. Most are centered around diet and skin care routines as follows:

Adults Don't Get Acne

Acne can affect people of all ages, but most acne products are designed for teenage or oily skin. This is where natural remedies and skin care products come in. You can make cleansers, moisturizers and treatments that effectively treat acne on an every day long term holistic basis. You can also save hundreds of dollars on skin care products when you make your own products at home.

Sunscreen Causes Acne

You can use sunscreen with acne, it won't make it worse but if you want to aid the clearing of pimples it is best to use a zinc oxide natural based cream that can actually help to heal skin.

Just Buy An Acne Wash

Many acne washes can be harsh on skin, especially for people with drier skin as most acne washes are designed for teenage or oily skins. The best solution is to make your own acne wash and other skin care products with antibacterial properties to cleanse and nourish your skin properly.

Chocolate And Candy Gives You Acne

While a healthy diet is important it's not necessarily the actual sugar that causes acne. Sugar does effect your hormones and metabolism, which has been shown to be related to acne breakouts, but direct consumption of sugar has not been directly associated with the cause of acne breakouts. Eating an alkaline diet in balance with an acid diet (eat your veggies people) does help to regulate hormones and sebum production. Consuming oils (like yummy salad dressings anyone?) that water down/increase the viscosity of your skins sebum will help to lubricate pores and aid their release of any hardened oil deposits. Good oils like almond and safflower or olive oils all help to loosen blocked pores from the inside and out especially when used in cleansers and serums.

Dairy products on the other hand have been debated widely for their acne causing influence. The jury is still out on this one, so if in doubt drink skim!

Using the wrong makeup or you can't wear it when you have a breakout

This is partially true, however, it's not what makeup you use, but HOW and when you remove it that counts. Night time while you sleep is when your skin repairs and renews itself. This is why it is important to cleanse your skin, removing oil, makeup and debris from your pores. You can use antibacterial cleansers followed by an antibacterial moisturizing lotion or serum to support the skins natural acne fighting processes.

Acne Is Caused By Poor Hygiene

A common assumption is that acne is caused by lack of personal hygiene. This is not true, however you can spread acne by rubbing, picking or scratching your skin. Washing your hands before washing your face is a good way to help prevent the spread of acne bacteria.

THE PSYCHOLOGICAL EFFECTS OF ACNE

Acne is one of the most prevalent skin conditions in adults and adolescents. For teenagers in the midst of the development of their self esteem, acne can have a very big impact. Studies have shown that the psychological effects of acne can lead to depression, social anxiety and withdrawal, or even eating disorders. Scarring is another issue that can leave a long term psychological impact. It is important to understand the methods (and recipes) you can use to prevent and protect skin from acne masks and scars.

Your skin is not you: it's only a part of you and need not be a permanent problem, just a small blip on the radar of your lifes journey. Taking small steps every day, you can deal with acne and prevent the lasting effects it can otherwise leave behind.

Severe acne may require medical intervention to treat it, but most of the time, you can take positive steps at home to treat and conceal acne and lessen its effects on your self esteem.

Small dietary changes can make a big difference to the frequency of acne breakouts. You don't need to take drastic action, by including a few small additions to your diet, like safflower or coconut oil for example, you can contribute to it's demise.

Topical concealers, available over-the-counter or by prescription are an option to hide blemishes. You can use concealers that contain tea tree or other essential oils (or even add a drop of these oils to your concealers but test that they do not coagulate them by mixing a drop of each together first). As a rule, avoid petroleum based products. There are many natural concealers on the market that you can find in our Amazon store at http://astore.amazon.com/bestp03b-20

If you are suffering from anxiety or depression, you may opt to visit a physician. Don't be afraid to seek help for your acne and any emotional problems that may be associated with it.

DETERMINING YOUR SKIN TYPE

Your skin type plays an important role in how acne affects you and also in how you should treat it. When it comes to acne, there is no one size fits all solution.

There are four basic skin types:

- Oily skin
- Normal skin
- Dry skin
- Dry skin
- Combination skin
- Mature skin

Skin changes over time and over different seasons. When targeting acne, teenage or oily skin does not need the same moisture treatment as dry skin. Obviously you don't want to strip the oil out of skin that is already dry. If you have oily skin on the other hand, the sound of applying greasy oily concoctions may feel "just wrong". Unfortunately the approach most acne product manufacturers take is - blast it with chemicals and remove any oil which is their "bazooka" method of dealing with acne.

Thankfully there are many ways to not only deal with acne but deeply nourish your skin with beneficial ingredients to lovingly care for all skin types leaving you with clear healthy blemish free skin.

Here Are Some Things To Consider

Is you skin oily, normal or dry? Do you have an oily T-zone along your forehead and down your nose with blackheads and congestion? If you have oily skin you are going to need a wash that loosens clogged material in pores, and for dry skin, a recipe that moisturizes your skin replacing lost hydration. If you have large pores, then a cleanser and moisturizer or steam that helps to clean and close pores is ideal.

How frequently do you breakout? Weekly, monthly, every few months? If it's monthly girls, the you can take evening primrose oil or natural supplements to help with hormone balance. If it's a teenage related issue, you can use cleansers that lessen the severity of acne and help to prevent or eliminate the type of environment where acne thrives.

Dry Skin

As a general rule, people with dry skin have fewer breakouts. They seldom have blackheads caused by excess oils buildup in skin. Dry skin usually has fewer visible pores but may suffer from lines and redness or red veins. Lighter skin is more likely to be dry than darker complexions. Dry skin forms wrinkles earlier than normal or oily skins and may burn in the sun (if light).

Normal Skin

People with normal skin and with combination skin usually suffer from occasional breakouts, sometimes from blackheads and enlarged pores in the "t-zone". It may feel dry after cleansing but not tight and will regain some of its moisture content over time.

Oily Skin

Oily skins tell another story. Oily skin is characterized by more frequent breakouts and the presence of enlarged pores and blackheads. Pores are usually quite visible, and skin may appear shiny and "wet". This skin type is less prone to wrinkles and stays youthful for longer. The (fixable) down side is that this skin type is often much more susceptible to acne problems.

Determining what type of skin you have means you can choose the best natural skin care recipe range of cleansers, moisturizers and treatments to suit your skin.

You can try many of the recipes in this book (or adapt them) to find the perfect recipes that feel great for your unique skin.

QUICK ACNE TIPS: DO'S AND DONT'S

The occasional acne breakout is inevitable, here are some tips for clearing it up fast and preventing damage or scarring. These are tips for what you should do and what you should avoid doing to avoid aggravating your acne.

Do:

Do keep your skin as clean as a whistle. Keep the affected area clean with natural cleansers, rinses or steams. Do use your treatments consistently and regularly. Take your medicine (or "an apple a day"), if taking oral antibiotics do not miss any doses or you could allow the acne bacteria to develop resistance and become ineffective.

Do try not to keep touching your face. Keep your fingers off!: Yes that means NO squeezing or picking!

Do use natural steams and recipes from this book and the acne scar prevention serums. They really help to make life impossible for the acne bacteria to stay, condition your skin, and maintain an environment where acne just feels unwelcome!

Do be cautious with OTC (over the counter) products. If you are going to use commercially made acne products, start with lower strength products. The point of this is to minimize redness, excessive dryness and other skin problems associated with these products. Try to gradually increase the strength and frequency of your applications over a fees weeks so your skin can adjust to the treatments.

Do use two products with different active ingredients to treat stubborn acne. Acne ingredients work in different ways, so you may find it helpful to use varying products and ingredients to treat stubborn acne. Apply one in the morning and the other at night to prevent skin irritation.

Be patient. It's possible that it's going to take a while to control your acne! Many people clear up their acne in days, but for some it can take a while to eliminate it for good. So be patient, it takes time but will happen! Learning what your skin likes may take two or three months of daily use of recipes (and a little experimentation with different recipes) to find the right system for you, but I promise, it will be worth it. Acne doesn't like being destroyed so remember it may briefly seem like it's getting worse before it gets better.

Do experiment with what works. You may need to try different recipes with varying active ingredients before you find a regimen that works for you (this applies especially to stubborn or severe acne).

Don't:

Don't pick! You've heard this before I know and I know its soooo tempting to pick and attack that zit. DON'T DO IT! No matter how tempting a good squeeze might be, leave it alone!

Can't resist? Use a tissue not your fingers or you will spread the nasty little bacteria sending out an invitation inviting it to stay.

Don't use petroleum oil products with ingredients like mineral oil or vaseline. They prolong the presence of bacteria on your skin.

Don't give up, use the tips and recipes in this book for at least a month, and you'll see a huge difference plus you'll ensure a long term result.

EFFECTIVE ACNE TREATMENT OPTIONS

Studies show that up to 70% of people from adults to teens suffer from some form acne sometime in their lives. There are many treatments, medicinal, natural and surgical to treat acne. Most are expensive and many have side effects or don't take into account your skin type. They are seen as short term treatments and are not something you can integrate into your skin care regime as a long term effective solution. Prevention through good skincare that you can make at home which contain antibacterial properties to deter acne bacteria from becoming established and make your skin an inhospitable place for acne bacteria to grow, is the key to clear skin for the long term.

Physicians and researchers have tried to find a "super treatment" for acne, but they all seem to focused on putting the fire out after it has started, not preventing it from starting in the first place.

Supplements, diet and good skincare can all contribute to clear skin, all of which you will be happy to read about in the following pages.

Current Acne Treatments

Drugs Or Medicated Washes

There are many acne treatments on the market. They all work in different ways. Some ingredients are formulated to target pustules and cysts while others try to eliminate the bacteria in the hair follicle to ensure the reduction and elimination of acne. Some products are intended for short term effect while others are designed with long-term results in mind.

The following are the most common ingredients used in acne products:

Isotretinoin

This ingredient can reduce oil or sebum production, soothes the inflammation in the form of pimples, pustules and cysts and can also help unblock the clogging of pores. However, use of this product can also produce side effects such as dryness and scaling of the skin, particularly on the lips.

Alcohol And Acetone

This is a mainstay ingredient in cleansers as well as astringent toners. Although these are effective in removing dirt and oils from the skin, they can cause a stinging or a burning sensation on the skin. If you have severe acne, it may be best to avoid these treatments (as advised by many dermatologists), however, it can prevent the increase of break-outs if you use them at the onset of acne.

Salicylic Acid

This ingredient is another fruit acid found in tomatoes and strawberries and also in willow bark (a natural tree bark powder you can buy from Amazon or health stores). The aim of salicylic acids is to dissolve comedones (blackheads) or whiteheads through the elimination of dead cells inside the hair follicles. This in turn prevents the pores from being clogged allowing oil or sebum to pass through without blockage. It can sting the first few times you use it and cause mild redness. Most products have a concentration of up to 2 percent salicylic acid in their preparation, however, for some people, a stronger mixture can be applied depending on your skin's needs. You can make salicylic acid masks to use at home using many of the recipes in this book (see the tomato strawberry mask).

Benzoyl Peroxide

This is one of the most common ingredients in acne products because it is considered to be the most active ingredient in acne treatment. It is essentially an anti-bacterial ingredient that helps remove bacteria in your follicles. It works by dissolving comedones (blackheads/blocked pores), an early sign of acne. Some products contain Benzoyl peroxide ratio of 2.5 to 10%, depending on the severity of your acne. This ingredients is recommended for early onset acne and for prevention. Side effects may include dryness and scaling in some people and redness and swelling in others. There are many natural alternatives like coconut oil, camellia essential oil, sandalwood and lemon essentials oils among others that can do this job just as effectively but without the irritation and with the added benefits of healing and repairing skin.

Alpha Hydroxy Acids

Glycolic acid and lactic acid are two common types of alpha hydroxy acids frequently used in OTC (over the counter) acne products. They are in fact the synthetic versions of acids derived from sugar-rich fruits (like many of the fruits included in recipes in this book). They treat acne by helping to remove dead skin cells and also by helping to reduce inflammation. Alpha hydroxy acids are also known to stimulate the growth of new, smoother skin, which helps reduce the appearance of acne scars.

Sulfur

This ingredient is rarely used alone as a product but rather included in acne products as an additional aid to reduce acne. Sulphur acts in a similar way to fruit acids by removing dead skin cells and excess oil. A keratolytic sulphur preparation may have a drying effect on the skin. It can cause initial irritation at the start of treatment. If this persists, it is advised that use of the product be discontinued or the strength reduced until the side effects subside.

Antibiotics

Some acne treatment products contain antibiotics to help kill bacteria and prevent the spread of acne. Some doctors may also prescribe antibiotics to help prevent scarring. Antibiotics (such as tetracycline, tretinoin and sodium sulfacetamide) are prescribed in oral or topical medications. They must be taken regularly and within the period prescribed. There are other "natural antibiotic" alternatives to taking these (again without side effects). For example a more natural remedy is tea tree oil which also has antibacterial properties and can be added to and applied in topical form like masks, oils, creams and gels. Honey is another "natural antibiotic" to use as a wonderful moisturizing healing and antibacterial base. You can make cleansers, masks and spot treatments from honey. In this book you will see the frequent use of tea tree oil for acne because it is so powerful and honey, because simply put - it kicks acne's butt when used together with other natural antibacterial ingredients like lavender oil, carrier oils which help to loosen and remove blackheads, and herbs.

Mild And Juvenile Acne

This kind of acne: is often described as teenage "zits". It can be effectively treated using over-the- counter (OTC) medicines available in most good drugstores. This kind of acne is considered to be amongst the easiest to treat but many prescription medical interventions are also effective as acne treatments. These include a range of antibiotics, adapalene, benzoylperoxide and tretinoin. These treatments help prevent or stunt the development of bacteria and decrease
   inflammation and reddening.

Depending on the person's skin type a doctor may choose to prescribe an acne treatment they believe to be appropriate and effective. As an example, if a patient has oily skin then certain creams and lotions would not be advisable, mainly as these are oil-based medications. Certain Gels and liquid solutions will be more suitable in this case since they are predominantly alcohol-based and therefore tend to dry out the skin. Most of the recipes in this book have similar properties and are just as effective.

Moderate To Severe Acne

If you acne has worsened over time characterized by an increased number of whiteheads and increased irritation or inflammation you may require a more advanced intervention.

Severe forms of acne may cover a larger area and may not be confined to the face but to the neck, back or other areas of the body. Dealing with acne severity may require a combination of oral medications such as tetracycline, minocycline, isotretinoin, doxycycline and erythromycin. (Erythromycin is the only pregnancy safe oral acne medicine).

These can cause side effects like upset stomach or other skin rashes. They can be used along with topical medications such as sulphur preparations that are known to be extremely effective as acne treatments. Sulphur loosens dead skin cells and removes them along with acne bacteria.

Understanding Teen Acne

Acne is most common in teenagers, and often impacts them psychologically as well as on their physical appearance. Teen acne is usually caused by increased hormonal activity within the skin's sebaceous glands. An increased level of oils mixed with dirt, makeup or blackheads (clogged pores) leads to lumps or lesions – what we call acne. The most common places for acne to occur is around the face, back, neck, buttocks, shoulders etc. This is where the oil glands are most concentrated making them the most problematic areas.

I am not going to cover the psychology of acne here, we all know it can have a huge impact on self esteem. My opinion is - the best way to solve the psychological effects of acne is just not to have it & just get rid of it - now!

Blackheads

You can remove blackheads by consuming oil like safflower oil or starflower oil to lubricate skin sebum from within (capsule or raw form in salad dressings etc). You can also use specific oils in cleansers to soften and dissolve the hardened sebum in clogged pores. If you are using a cleanser that isn't one I recommend in this book (commercially produced), avoid using products that contain alcohol, mineral oil or petroleum-based additives. These ingredients and others like sodium laureth sulphate or sodium lauryl sulphate can be very harsh, strip skin and often make the problem worse.

Sulphates in particular can strip the skin of its natural acid mantle (otherwise known as the natural emollients and oils produced by your skin). Stripping these oils away also over stimulates the glands in an effort to replace the "lost oil". Products containing natural oils and ingredients are less likely to block pores, and are much gentler to the skin. Sulphates are also found in shampoo, hand and body washes. They can also damage eye membranes, especially in children.

You can also use gentle exfoliants to remove excess skin cells, oils and grime but be careful not to rub and aggravate irritated skin. Avoid squeezing blackheads and spreading bacteria further around skin.

Back Acne: Causes And Treatments

Back acne pustules and pimples can be more persistent compared to facial acne. This is because the skin is in constant contact with clothing which encourages oil production and the spread of acne bacteria through rubbing.

Glycolic acid body washes are great for back acne, especially with the addition of tea tree oil as they combat acne bacteria and remove the excessive oils without drying out the skin.

Cystic Acne: Causes And Treatment

Cystic acne, as the name suggests, forms as a cyst under the skin and can be quite painful. It is large and unsightly and can scar if squeezed and picked. It is essentially an inflammation of the follicle and the surrounding tissue which may grow into cystic nodules filled with pus that is tender to the touch.

The most common treatment for cystic acne is a drug known as 'Accutane', an oral medication usually prescribed over a course of 20 weeks. It works by slowing the production of oil and interrupting the environment bacteria grows in. It is also known to help prevent scarring. Many natural remedies also do this.

Despite it's significant cost, unfortunately many people do not complete their full course of accutane and find that their acne returns often worse than before. It also can include side effects like abnormal liver enzymes, dry mouth, skin and nose, itchy skin, sore muscles, inflamed eye and mouth membranes. It also effects cholesterol, triglyceride and lipid levels in your body. Pregnant women should never take this drug as it can cause birth defects.

Salon Treatments Offered For Acne

Here are a range of some of the modern acne treatments offered by salons:

Acne Facials

Salon treatments for acne include acne facials for acne afflicted problematic skin. Many procedures involve steam vapor mists, enzymatic or glycolic acid exfoliation, deep pore cleansing, electronic treatments and anti-bacterial masks.

Microdermabrasion

MicroDermabrasion is used mainly for removal of scarring and discoloration. Treatments usually last half to a whole hour and leave your skin red for a period of time up to 24 hours afterwards.

The Oxyjet Anti-Acne Treatment

The OXYjet Anti-Acne Treatment is one of the latest skin rejuvenation treatments around. It utilizes the latest biotechnology to get remove flaws and blemishes, fight bacteria and help to restore hormonal balance. They are usually performed every few months and can be expensive.

Bio Oxygen Anti-Aging Treatments

Bio Oxygen anti-aging deep pore treatments are salon treatments that work by gently pushing oxygen and effective cosmetic formulations deep into the skin with the use of a no-needle injection by way of a pressurized jet of oxygen. Again this can be expensive.

Light Therapy

Light therapy is quick, painless and inexpensive system that works by emitting blue light wavelengths into your skin. These waves are naturally anti- inflammatory, and can improve circulation. They also help cleanse follicles and glands by destroying acne bacteria and by soothing and balancing oil production.

Isotretinoin And Panthothenate Gardena Treatments

These are two types of acne treatments that use Isotretinoin or d-calcium panthothenate. These are oral treatments and work by reducing oil production in the skin. Isotretinoin can make acne worse for a short period before it gets better, just something to be aware of.

More About Doctor Prescribed Acne Medications

For people suffering from acute or prolonged acne, over the counter medicines are not enough. Sometimes it many be necessary to seek doctor prescribed acne medicines. These kinds of medication, both oral and topical, can be more effective than over the counter medicines.

Types Of Prescription Medicines:

Antibiotics

Antibiotics commonly used to combat acne can be taken orally or applied topically as a lotion. Topical prescription medications may include ingredients like zinc to help healing or retinoids (vitamin A derivative) to speed the healing process and prevent or repair scarring. There are of course many natural sources of vitamin A including carrot seed oil which is an excellent ingredients to add to your own acne recipes.

The most commonly utilized antibiotic used for treating acne is tetracycline. This kills the bacteria responsible for acne and also reduces inflammation. A common side effect associated with tetracycline is increased sensitivity to sun light, dizziness, yeast infections (I'm talking to you ladies) hives, and also an upset stomach. Treatment may take several weeks or even months and a full course must be completed for it to be effective.

Antibiotics also have side effects and taking them for a prolonged period of time over several courses can reduce their effectiveness. So even though you may have to take them for many months, they can eventually become ineffective as the bacteria develop resistance to the antibiotic or intolerable because of common side effects like stomach upsets, recurring yeast infections and other skin problems (some worse than acne itself).

Topical Antibiotic Acne Treatments Include The Following:

- Clindamycin
- Metronidazole
- Erythromycin
- Minocycline
- Tetracycline

Again these can cause dizziness, nausea and vomiting, must be taken for a long period of time and can become resistant especially if you don't take them consistently or finish the full course.

Ointments And Topical Solutions

Antibiotic ointments generally come with fewer complications than oral antibiotics yet are effective in killing bacteria that cause. You can use antibiotic treatments along side other topical treatments like benzoyl peroxide which helps prevent the bacteria developing a resistance to the antibiotics. I prefer of course to use natural alternatives that are just as effective or potent on your skin. Ingredients like tea tree oil, neem oil, honey (UMF active honey) and spices like turmeric powder work astoundingly well together as an effective treatment. You can add these to everyday moisturizers as well (yes I'm going to show you how to make those).

Retinoids

Retinoids are a form of acne medication derived from vitamin A. They can can be applied directly to the skin typically in the form of a cream or lotion. They help to remove dead layers of skin, unclog pores and loosen congestion.

Oral retinoids are the next step up and are used for more severe forms of acne. Unfortunately side effects of taking oral retinoids can also cause liver damage and depression and should NOT be taken while pregnant.

Corticosteroids

These are the big (scary) guns for treating acne and can only be taken for a very short time. We've all heard about the effects of steroids on our bodies – so this is a last resort short term option for people who have exhausted all other avenues of treatment.

Birth Control

Some birth control pills are prescribed to help regulate hormone imbalances thus reducing the acne causing effects of testosterone.

Accutane

Accutane is a prescription drug for the treatment of very severe cystic or nodular acne. This is usually prescribed as a last resort. Again it can have unpleasant side effects and is not good for your liver.

Acne Home Treatments

This is the section you have been waiting for. It's where the fun begins and you get down to business and begin the process of eliminating your acne.

This is where you get to make your own acne recipes, "play with" different home treatments and discover skin care lotions, cleansers and more that will not only clear your acne but nourish and feed your skin.

Remember, your skin is unique to you, and you are going to have a lot of recipes to choose from, so you can pick what works for you. I have designed these recipes so that you can use them long term, and incorporate them into your skin care routine.

This isn't just an acne recipe book, it's also an introduction to making your own skin care products. Although you will be using acne eliminating ingredients in these recipes, you can reduce their concentrations once you have your acne under control. You can lower the active acne treatment ingredients, and add in scar reducing ingredients like rose hip and carrot seed oils instead.

The reason why this system is so effective is that it allows you to gently move from one phase to another of your acne treatment, all the while supporting and nourishing your skin giving it exactly what it needs to look and feel it's best.

So let's get to it!

Doing It Yourself

As we have just discussed, treating your acne doesn't need to involve buying a bunch of expensive prescriptions or even over-the-counter products.

The beauty of using natural treatments is that they are designed not only to deal with your acne issue as fast and immediately as any commercial treatment, but also for the long term.

Acne can be a long term thing IF you focus only on the immediate area (the current "generation" of acne bacteria) and not the systemic cause of it.

If you weed the garden, but don't take out the seeds or bulbs, you'll just have a flourishing mess of new weeds to deal with a few weeks later.

The same thing applies to your skin. Acne washes and treatments are designed for a specific use for a specific time period. Or for a specific skin type (which may not be yours).

If you were to use acne washes and treatments long term;

A it's often expensive and

B your skin is missing out on all of the other nutrients it needs in the mean time.

Why not make your own skin care products that feed and nurture your skin AND also treat and prevent acne making your skin an inhospitable rather than welcoming place for acne to reside.

HOW ACNE TREATMENTS WORK

Herbal acne remedies work in several ways to cleanse pores, balance hormones which regulate sebum production, and lubricate (or water down) your body's natural sebum so it is more viscose and able to be excreted more readily from pores.

They also help to change the environment acne likes to thrive in making your skin a less hospitable environment for acne bacteria to grow in.

They also help to support your body's ability to eliminate toxins.

As you read on about ingredients and recipes, you'll discover what each ingredient does to combat acne or support and heal your skin.

Paleo And Alkaline Diets

These diets have been shown to help with acne related issues. This is thought to be because the foods that these diets limit can impact on your hormones through regulating the sugar and acid balance in your body thus eliminating some of the factors that encourage acne bacteria growth.

Skin Exfoliation Treatments For Acne

There are two different types of exfoliation you can perform on skin to help with acne. Physical and chemical.

Physical acne treatments involve granular pastes made of husks, beads or grains. These work by sloughing off or dissolving dead skin cells. Chemical exfoliators are acid based and contain active ingredients like salicylic or other fruit acids, enzymes which peel away the top layers of skin. You can use these two exfoliation types separately or combined.

You can also make your own acne exfoliators using strawberries, tomatoes, tea tree or other essential oils and brown sugar or salt depending on your skin type.

Over The Counter Acne Remedies

If making pastes and extracts just isn't your cup of tea, there are many over the counter options you can buy or from online stores.

You can also add a few drops of tea tree oil (up to 5%) to your usual facial wash or cleanser and rinse your skin with an almond oil, coconut oil, lemon juice and tea tree cleanser in the shower for a quick antibacterial moisturizing treatment.-

Washing your skin removes excess oils that may build up and clog your pores.

Acne OTC Topical Treatments

If you walk down the aisle of your local drug store or supermarket looking for an acne product, you'll see no shortage of options.

Most OTC washes and creams will have Benzyl peroxide in them or salicylic acid, common antibacterial ingredients that are designed to remove oils and dirt from skin and treat acne bacteria at the same time. They also help to stop the further spread of acne around the skin.

For these products to be effective, you will need to use them on a regular basis as directed by the manufacturer.

You can buy tea tree based natural washes like those found in our online Amazon store. These are generally a lot less harsh on skin and reactions to the active ingredients in these products are also much less likely. If you have dry or sensitive skin these are a great option.

You can of course make your own products at home very simply and without hassle. You don't need to be a cosmetic lab technician to formulate and make these recipes, if you can mix pancakes – you can make your own skin care products!

Other topical acne treatments like Clindamycin (a topical antibiotic) can be obtained in lotion, solution or even gel formulations at around 1% strength.

Tetracycline (a sulfur and sodium extract based product) is another topical treatment that is becoming popular.

These need to be applied twice a day to be effective and can irritate skin especially with prolonged use.

It is always advisable to consult your doctor regarding the best treatment for your acne rather than experimenting with OTC drugs.

Natural "Antibiotic" Alternative Treatments

There are many "natural antibiotics" in nature which can have a very positive effect on your body's ability to deal with acne itself – from the inside as well as out.

Ingredients like:

- UMF honey (active honey) offers a strong natural defense against bacteria. Take (eat) a teaspoon (or two) daily of UMF 16+ (from a health store on Amazon) honey as an internal antimicrobial medicine.
- Colloidal silver has been known to effectively target "bad" bacteria in your gut and throughout your whole body.
- Echinacea is great (in tablet form) as is Olive leaf extract to counteract acne bacteria
- Yogurt with a high level of acidophilus, bifidus and other "good" bacteria (fights the "bad" guys). Take a Tbsp a day or add it to smoothies to support your body's natural balance. If you have or are trying acne antibiotic medicines make sure you replace the good

bacteria any antibiotics destroy with a regular intake of yogurt.

Oral Acne Treatments

Oral acne treatments are generally only prescribed for people with acute acne, and other options are available like the contraceptive pill Diane which contains an ingredient 'cyproterone acetate' which is known to be effective in counteracting acne.

Food Sensitivities

Recent studies have shown that food sensitivities to foods such as such seafood, wheat, dairy and fruits may contribute to acne. A study conducted recently deduced that that women consuming three or more glasses of milk per day were 22% more likely to have acne breakouts than women consuming only one glass of milk per day.

Some say this is due to the hormone levels present in milk, others because it changes the composition or consistency of the serum in your skin making it more susceptible to becoming "stuck" or blocked in pores.

High acid foods have also been shown to have a potential effect on the frequency and amplitude of acne breakouts.

No matter what the theorists conclude, a balanced alkaline biased diet seems to be the consistent winner in the debate over what foods or food allergies/sensitivities have the most impact on your skin as far as acne is concerned. The vast majority of people who eat vegetables or some sort of greens and raw food on a regular basis, seem to have better clearer skin.

Treating Cystic Acne

Cystic acne is generally considered to be the most severe form of acne vulgaris. It begins from very deep with the pores of your skin originating from a congested area that has become infected. Cystic acne has the appearance of a nodule but can be filled with pus with a diameter of 5mm or more. The lesions formed can very tender and painful. They can also leave scarring especially if disturbed.

Cystic Acne Treatments

There needs to be a three pronged approach when targeting cystic acne to ensure it's effective treatment. Clearing the pores and changing the environment for acne lesions to form, treating the bacteria itself and removing all traces of it from the existing areas so it cannot spread, and preventing scarring .

Some Treatments For Cystic Acne Include:

A medical physician draining the area or in extreme cases surgical extraction

Blue light therapy to neutralize bacteria

Laser therapy to "blast" the bacteria and lighten scars

Accutane treatment to regulate sebaceous glands

Cortisone injections to the effected sites to reduce swelling and infection

Isotretinoin prescription to help stop scarring

Oral contraceptives like Diane to reduce hormone imbalances

These can be fairly invasive or extreme, and may be necessary but with the right natural treatments (from the inside and out) you shouldn't need them.

More About Medical Advice

Ask your doctor what options there are if you need to, but remember some treatments may not work the first time. You can use many different drugs, but many are not long term solutions and can have significant side effects. Surgical Options

Often, when every avenue of medicinal treatment is exhausted, there comes a time for sufferers of persistent acne or more severe acne to seek alternative treatment methods. A dermatologist can help discuss the different treatments currently available including treating acne with laser therapy or acne surgery.

If you are considering the possibility of treating acne with laser therapy or surgery, you must take care to fully evaluate each of the processes, including the number of required treatments, the consequent costs, and the potential side effects of the treatment. It's also important that you select a process that is designed to deal with reducing the presence of acne, and not just acne scarring.

Acne Surgery

Acne surgery involves making an incision into the affected area and draining the clogged matter. The process for blackheads and whiteheads doesn't actually involve surgery, but is often performed by a nurse, esthetician or dermatologist. A small, pointed blade is used to first open the comedone and then gently work the material out using a comedone extractor.

Severe cysts can be drained and removed by a procedure known as excisional surgery. The procedure should be performed in a sterile environment to reduce the risk of spreading bacterial infection and should only be performed by trained professional. If the cysts are not carefully extracted, they can develop serious infection and create scarring.

PHYSICAL TREATMENTS

Exfoliation

This form of treatment involves removing the top layer of skin either chemically or with some sort of abrasive. Chemical peels are usually done with salicylic acid or glycolic acid. These work by destroying a microscopic layer of skin cells to unclog pores and remove the build-up of dead cells. The same effect can be achieved by using an abrasive cloth or liquid scrub.

Comedone Extraction And Drainage

This procedure involves application of an anesthetic cream to the immediate area of breakout. Blackheads and white heads are then extracted using a pen-like instrument which opens the head and allows removal of the contents of the pore. A topical antibiotic cream is normally applied pot procedure.

Drainage is essential the same thing but may involve needle extraction (sounds lovely right?).

Laser Treatments

Laser resurfacing is one of the most popular treatments for many scar related skin disorders. The most well-known laser types used in laser resurfacing of acne scars are the carbon dioxide (CO_2) and erbium:YAG (Er:YAG) lasers.

These used pulsed light waves to remove the surface layers of skin, reduce overly-large sebaceous glands and acne lesions stimulating new cell growth and healthy skin. Laser treatments remove the damaged outer layers of skin to stimulate new cell growth.

Laser treatments can be expensive, there are natural alternatives like homemade peels that do a similar job, without the expense or down time.

Essential Oils

The best acne treatments are not necessarily the well known and marketed acne medications that contain chemicals. Other effective acne treatments include essential oils, which can be applied topically for acne conditions ranging from mild to moderate. One of the best acne treatments when it comes to essential oils is tea tree oil.

Tea tree oil is highly antibacterial, making it an effective acne treatment. Tea tree oil belongs to the best acne treatments group because it efficiently soothes irritation, prevents and controls acne. It is widely regarded as one of the best acne treatments because it is fast acting and works quickly to clear up the skin while soothing the affected area.

NATURAL SOLUTIONS FOR ACNE AND GORGEOUS CLEAR SKIN

Now for the best part…..

You are looking for a final solution to your to your acne and blemish issues. You want clear, unblemished healthy skin.

You can make a huge range of all natural treatments from herbs, fruits, spices etc. that you probably already have around your house. With the addition of essential oils, your recipes will become a multi faceted acne destroying (and skin nurturing) skin transforming tool kit.

You will be able to try a variety of cleansers, rinses, steams, pastes, and facial masks made from different natural ingredients.

Using simple ingredients like vinegar, salt, lemon, turmeric, you can clean skin and remove excess skin oils. Lemon, lime, or tomato juice are great with honey for a cleanser.

Fruits contain fruit acids to help reduce acne bacteria. Potassium in bananas and avocados retards acne bacteria. Tropical fruits like pineapple or papaya contain enzymes to dissolve dead skin cells and blackheads.

Honey (especially UMF active honey) is a natural antibiotic, so is colloidal silver and tea tree oil, and coconut oil.

Herbs and herbal products including cinnamon, neem bark, willow bark, basil, mint, rosemary, thyme, turmeric, and nutmeg can be made into a solution or paste and used as well.

Oatmeal and chamomile and cucumber soothe itchy or red inflamed skin. Lavender essential oil calms redness and irritation.

Essential oils like myrrh, tea tree, neem, lavender, rosemary, sandalwood, fenugreek and manuka are antibacterial and antimicrobial and soothing.

Many skin care cleansers, moisturizers and masks can be made from these ingredients and others like glycerin, almond oil, rose hip, carrot seed and many other oils to deeply nourish and repair skin.

You can add many of the "active" ingredients above to your lotions and recipes to make a powerful recipe that is perfect for YOUR skin type.

More simple common sense advice:

- Drink plenty of water every day.
- Eat lots of omega3 fatty acids I supplement in fresh form (oils, fish, salad dressings).
- Take a break from processed preservative and coloring laden foods and watch what happens. Not only will you feel better but your skin will look better too.
- On that note, go organic as much as humanly possible. The fewer chemicals you put in (or on) your body, the clearer your skin will most likely be.
- Consider taking vitamin A and zinc supplements – these ingredients help skin also.
- Try organic foods and products where you can...give it a go for a month.

Time To Give Your Acne It's Final Eviction Notice

Natural acne skin care is the answer to LONG TERM clear skin. That's what the next chapter is all about...

INGREDIENTS

Start with the right ingredients, once you know what you can use, you'll learn how to use them...

The following ingredients are beneficial for Acneic skin:

- Almond meal
- Aloe vera
- Apple
- Apple cider vinegar
- Apricots raw
- Arrowroot
- Basil
- Bergamot
- Calendula
- Carrot seed oil
- Cucumber
- Eucalyptus
- Evening primrose oil
- Frankincense
- Fruits (especially tomatoes, strawberries, papaya and apple)
- Gotu kola
- Guava
- Herbs
- Honey
- Juniper
- Lavender oil
- Macadamias
- Manuka oil
- Milk
- Neem oil
- Orange
- Oatmeal
- Pomegranate
- Rosehip oil
- Tea tree oil
- Turmeric

- Vitamin A.
- Yoghurt

Turmeric

When it comes to home-made acne treatments, turmeric is one of the most simple yet effective ingredients. Turmeric is famous for its ability to nourish the skin and to eliminate facial scars. For oily skin, turmeric home-made acne treatments can be made by combining it with rose water to make paste. Another effective combination is a mixture of turmeric and lemon juice.

Honey

Honey is another naturally anti-bacterial and anti-microbial important ingredient in home-made acne treatments. It can be used as a facial that's applied directly or mixed with lemon juice or essential oils. Honey-apple as a combination is also one of the most well-known home-made acne treatments.

Fresh Fruits And Vegetables

Home-made acne treatments also involve fresh fruits and vegetables, which may be in sliced or in paste form. Most commonly used home-made acne treatments include potato and cucumber, which are sliced in round shapes and placed on the face. Grape juice and orange juices are also popular home-made acne treatments as they contain fruit acids to combat acne.

Baking Soda

Home-made acne treatments like baking soda mask also help fight acne. After washing your face using a mild cleanser, mix a little baking soda with water and apply gently on your face. This mixture helps clear your acne aside from making it soft and clear.

Oatmeal

Other home-made acne treatments include oatmeal. To make an oatmeal mask, blend a little oatmeal with water. Gently apply on your skin and leave it on for 15 minutes. Oatmeal masks are gentle and safe. They are also great home-made acne treatments because they soothe and heal skin. Make a thick paste with oatmeal and warm water, apply on the affected area, leave it on for 20 minutes, and then rinse with warm water. This is especially effective for those with regular acne and acne rosacea.

There are also home-made acne treatments that relieve redness and itching. Make a baking soda paste and apply it on the problem area. While this is more popularly known as a bee sting relief rather than one of the home-made acne treatments, it also lessens itching and redness in acne sufferers.

Acne Natural Treatments

Natural acne products (made at home by you or store bought) are an ideal alternative to commercial products because they do not contain the high levels of chemicals that can produce reactions and side effects. Natural acne solutions attack the problem in several ways to provide the most thorough and comprehensive treatment possible.

What Options Are There?

What you consume and also what you apply to your body are both important for regulating the factors that encourage or help prevent acne. Eating a well balanced diet, one that is rich in vitamins and minerals is a great start. Next you can use natural but effective topical treatments from masks to serums and cleansers to clean and protect your skin.

Here are some types of supplements that may be able to help you fight acne:

Zinc

Zinc Vitamin is a natural element that you need in your diet every day. It has been shown to be effective at treating inflammatory acne. It may not be as beneficial as some of the medications, both oral and topical, that you can use, but it does help when trying to avoid these products.

Chromium

Chromium supplement has been shown to help in some cases as well.

Safflower Oil, Starflower Oil

These help to lubricate the sebum so pores do not get blocked or congested as easily.

Evening Primrose Oil

A hormone balancing oil that regulates your system – a balancing oil.

Multi-Vitamins

In many ways, a good multi-vitamin can offer overall help to you too.

You can even find combinations specifically for acne.

Natural supplements support your body's balance and ability to fight acne naturally.

Olive Leaf Extract

Helps to support the liver and immune system.

Herbal Cortisone

A natural alternative to synthetic cortisones.

Tea Tree Oil Cream

Tea tree oil (as I have already said and will say many times again), is natures natural bacteria blasting wonder product. It is antibacterial, antibacterial and antimicrobial. I use it for many of my acne remedies – well most actually! And that's because it packs such a mighty punch. Honey's soothing, moisturizing and healing powers (also antimicrobial) tone tea tree down so that when you use the two ingredients together, they work synergistically to combat acne and heal skin at the same time.

CLEAR SKIN FROM THE INSIDE OUT

Nutrition plays a big part in skin health. Eating a diet rich in essential fatty acids and eating less acid producing foods can make a big difference. Below you will find some easy salad dressing recipes you can make as a way to get "good" oils into your body. These help to lubricate your oils sebum and help reduce the likelihood of clogged pores which encourage pimples.

Salad Dressing Recipes

You can make your own dressings that contain beneficial or "good oils" for your skin and general health. Consuming fatty acids in your diet like fish oils, safflower and other fatty acids, helps your skin maintain healthy sebum levels while lowering your cholesterol. Most plant-based oils are low in saturated fat but there are oils such as palm and coconut oils which are high in saturated and fats and therefore should be avoided.

Monounsaturated Fatty Acids

Olive, canola and peanut oil are high in monounsaturated fatty acids, which may lower your total and LDL cholesterol levels.

Polyunsaturated Fatty Acids

Polyunsaturated fatty acids are known to be heart-healthy. They contain sources of vitamin E and make a good choice for a salad dressing. Oils high in polyunsaturated fats are:

- Corn oil
- Safflower oil
- Sunflower oil

- Soybean oils

If you are purchasing an oil-based salad dressing, you can check the label to ensure that it doesn't contain trans fats from partially hydrogenated oils

Flaxseed Oil

Flaxseed oil is the most concentrated source of alpha-linolenic acid, an essential omega-3 fatty acid. Other sources of omega-3 fatty acids are walnuts or oily fish, such as tuna or salmon.

Recipes For Salad Dressings

Making salad dressings and vinaigrettes are easy. You can come up with your own basic dressings using the oils above with some of the ingredients below:

- Mustard
- Garlic
- Lime
- Lemon
- Balsamic vinegar
- Coriander
- Basil or other fresh herbs
- Sugar
- Paprika
- Chilli
- Parmesan cheese
- Parsley
- Pepper
- Almond slithers
- Sesame seeds
- Apple cider vinegar (great for skin)
- Tomato

- Fresh cream
- Yoghurt
- Cucumber
- Mint
- Egg yolks (whisk in to oil drop by drop to make a creamy dressing)
- Pine nuts
- Walnuts
- Pumpkin seeds

BASIC OIL DRESSING BASE (Add Your Own Additives To Taste)

The Vinaigrette Formula

The basic ratio of oil to vinegar when making vinaigrettes is 3 to 1. All you need to remember is three parts oil to one part vinegar and you'll have a good foundation for delicious dressings.

You can add creamy ingredients or eggs to make creamy dressings with a hint of sugar to enhance or sweeten the taste.

The secret is to mix a basic formula using one of the oils above and then slowly whisk in vinegar and any other ingredients. Flavors develop over time after sitting for a while leaving a dressing to rest in the fridge will bring out the flavor. Keep this in mind when adding herbs & spices, its easy to add too much.

You can test the flavor of your vinaigrette by dipping a piece of lettuce into your mixture, shaking off the excess and then taking a bite. Add more ingredients to taste.

Here are some delicious recipes to get you started:

Base Salad Dressing Mix

1 cup of extra virgin olive oil (or safflower oil, sunflower oil, or any of the oils above)

- 1 cup of white wine vinegar
- A dash of salt and pepper

Whisk together in a bowl before adding fresh ingredients and allow to sit for at least 1 an hour

Raspberry Vinaigrette

- 1 cup of raspberries: fresh or frozen
- 1 cup of vegetable oil
- 1 cup of apple cider vinegar
- 1 cup of balsamic vinegar
- 2 tsps of sugar
- 1 tsp of dijon mustard
- Herbed vinaigrette salad dressing

To your standard vinaigrette base, add 1 Tbsp Dijon mustard, 2 Tbsp chopped parsley, 1 tsp of your favorite dried herbs (such as thyme, basil, or marjoram) and whisk together well.

Mustard Flavored Salad Dressing (Mustard Vinaigrette)

- 1 Tbsp dijon mustard
- To make honey dijon add 1 Tbsp honey to the mustard vinaigrette

Italian And Asian Styled Salad Dressings

- For an italian vinaigrette, start with the base dressing and add

- 1 tsp minced garlic
- 1 tsp of dried oregano and
- 1 Tbsp chopped parsley

Asian Vinaigrette Dressing (Use Rice Vinegar)

- 1 Tbsp soy sauce
- 2 Tbsp sesame oil
- 1 Tbsp fresh minced or grated ginger
- 1 clove minced garlic
- A hint of chili sauce

Allow to sit for at least 30 minutes to allow the flavors to blend together.

Lime And Olive Oil Dressing

I like to whisk this right in the salad bowl and then just put the salad on top and toss.

- 1 Tbsp lime juice (from a bottle is fine)
- 1 Tbsp water
- 2 Tbsp extra virgin olive oil

Add lime juice and water to a bowl, then salt and pepper. Whisk in Olive oil then add seasoning and sweetener to taste.

Raita (Delicious Dressing And Face Mask Too)

Raita is a cold yogurt condiment that is often served with Indian food to balance the heat of the spicy dishes. It's good to eat and as a face mask.

- 1 large unpeeled cucumber, halved, seeded, coarsely grated
- 2 cups plain whole-milk yogurt

- 1 cup (packed) chopped fresh mint
- 1 tsp ground cumin
- 1 tsp plus pinch of cayenne pepper

Wrap grated cucumber in kitchen towel and squeeze dry. Whisk yogurt, mint, cumin, and 1 tsp cayenne pepper in a bowl to blend. Add cucumbers and toss to coat.

Add salt and pepper to taste. Cover and refrigerate for at least 2 hours. Omit cayenne pepper if you are using this recipe for a face mask.

Tzatziki Dip/Dressing (Also Good As A Cooling Exfoliating Face Mask)

A cool and creamy tangy cucumber dip flavored with garlic, it perfectly compliments grilled meats and vegetables. It's served on the side with warm pita bread triangles for dipping. Goes well with souvlaki.

- 3 Tbsp olive oil
- 1 Tbsp vinegar
- 2 cloves garlic, minced finely
- 1 tsp salt
- 1 tsp white pepper
- 1 cup greek yogurt, strained
- 1 cup sour cream
- 2 cucumbers, peeled, seeded and diced
- 1 tsp chopped fresh dill

Combine olive oil, vinegar, garlic, salt, and pepper in a bowl until well combined. Whisk the yogurt together with the sour cream then add the olive oil mixture to the yogurt mixture and mix well. Lastly, add the cucumber and chopped fresh dill. Refrigerate for at least two hours before serving.

Nutty Dressings

You can add ground or chopped nuts to a dressing to make it extra tasty and crunchy or finely chopped herbs.

These are just a few basic recipes to start with. You can create your own anytime you like using the beneficial oils described in this book for healthier skin and body.

Green Smoothies

One of the quickest, and least painful ways to give your skin and body a pep up is with green smoothies. Check out our website for some wondrous recipes for your skin and general health…YUM YUM!!

Makeup Fast

Eeeek no makeup? Got you! I'm not going to tell you not to wear makeup – just make sure you wash it off before bed so your pores can breathe and not tuck the little bacteria nasties into bed with a nice warm blanket (by not washing off the layer of grime that keeps them in). Wash skin well before bed and nourish your skin.

Work Out For Good Skin

Do something – get moving whether it's a walk, run, swim, jump on the trampoline or wrestling with a kid…it all helps get your circulation going and helps to stimulate your glands into moving that gunge out of your pores. Again wash your skin after exercise to remove dirt grime and oil.

De-Stress Your Face

Yoga, reading, nature – anything that de-stresses you DO it! It will help your skin and your soul ☺

Stuff To Put Your Face For Acne And Oily Skin

Activated charcoal

Aloe vera gel

Apple Cider Vinegar

Argan oil

Baking Soda

Basil

Buttermilk

Cabbage Leaves

Calendula marigold flowers

Carrots

Chamomile

Cosmetic clay kaolin bentonite French green rhassoul fuller's earth

Cucumber

Egg Whites

Essential oils lavender rosemary neem basil tea tree lemon peppermint

Evening primrose oil

Fennel

Garlic

Green Tea

Honey (UMF active honey is best)

Jojoba oil

Lemon Juice

Lime Juice

Neem oil or powder

Orange Peel

Papaya

Peppermint

Plain Yogurt

Potatoes

Red Wine

Rosemary

Sage

Sea Salt

Spinach

Strawberries

Tamanu oil

Tomatoes

Turmeric

Witch Hazel

Combine these foods with the essential oils or spices to make an extra potent facial treatment. Used on a regular basis they will transform your skin, especially when added to skin care moisturizers and lotions.

Most of these items can be found at a natural foods store (Whole Foods for example) or ordered online from Amazon or Mountain Rose Herbs.

You can also try recipes with one ingredient, well its not really a recipe, but rubbing a potato on your face or dusting some arrowroot powder on your skin then rinsing it off can control oiliness for a few hours.

Cleansing Your Skin With Oil

As an oily skinned person (yes you're who I am talking to) I'm hearing you say "what are you crazy?"...don't roll your eyes or go into shock at this point if you have oily skin and you're thinking I'm completely mad for telling you to clean your skin with oil?

The fact is – when you remove or strip too much oil from your skin (because you think you have too much of it), your body goes into oil replacement production overdrive. If you have oily skin that's prone to blackheads it's obviously very good at producing sebum, and so if you start removing it – it will get to work and make a whole lot more to replace it! This blocks pores and you end up with pimples. Makes sense huh!

The thing is – if you use the RIGHT oils (highest purest quality fast absorbing essential fatty acids rich oils) mixed with pure essential oils, you can dissolve or dilute the oils that clog pores and clear out the impurities that lead to pimples.

You skin will take a little time to get used to oil based cleansers, but there are some things you can do to reduce or eliminate the feeling of oily skin after you have used them, so don't worry, you're not going to be left with a face that feels like a fried food restaurant's kitchen after a Saturday night.

Oils offer many benefits for skin. Oils rich in essential fatty acids (EFA's) are easily and rapidly absorbed by your skin and in doing so deliver benefits (antibacterial bacteria fighting and healing properties) deep into the deeper layers of your skin where they can do their work fighting acne bacteria.

Oils like almond and wheat germ are great carrier oils as is coconut oil which is on it's own full of antibacterial properties. These oils dissolve the oil that clogs pores and encourages pimples.

Add to these tea tree, lavender and carrot seed oil with a pinch of turmeric powder for a potent acne cleanser.

You can go one step further and mix these with beeswax, honey, aloe vera and optional glycerin for a super hydrating creamy non oily acne cleanser with added healing properties.

Give these recipes a go and you'll change the way you look at your skin and the products you use. Simple is good – if you know what to use and how to use it.

Oil-Based Cleansing Methods

Here is a simple base recipe to use that you can change and adapt depending on your skin type and what you have available around home.

- Mix together 1 Tbsp of cold pressed castor or coconut oil with a carrier oil like jojoba, almond grapeseed, sesame, or hazelnut oil at a ratio of 2 parts castor/coconut oil to 1 part carrier oil.
- Next add 5 drops of lavender, tea tree and optionally neem oil. Mix them all together well.

- You can add a tsp of honey for it's extra healing and moisturizing qualities if you wish at this point. Honey doesn't like mixing with oil so you'll have to stir well before application or add a little arrowroot powder or ground oatmeal. You can also add a squeeze of lemon or lime juice if you have very oily skin (or apple cider vinegar).
- Dampen your skin with a splash of water or warm facecloth.
- Rub the mixture over your whole face and décolletage for several minutes. If you have time, place a warm wash cloth over your face to allow the oils to absorb easily for around 20 to 30 seconds.
- Wash this mixture off wiping well with the cloth until you have removed all excess oil.
- Your skin should feel soft and not oily after a few minutes.

At this point you an use a follow up toner (see toner recipes) or alternatively use a scrub instead if you have a lot of flakiness and your skin feels like it needs a good scrub.

Gentle Daily Acne And Oily Skin Face Scrub

- 1/2 cup finely ground oats
- 1 Tbsp brown sugar
- 1 Tbsp honey
- ½ cup finely ground raw organic sunflower seeds or raw almonds
- ½ cup organic white rice flour
- 1 tsp rock salt finely ground
- 10 drops lavender, tea tree, neem and/or pink grapefruit essential oil
- 1 tsp finely chopped basil leaves, mint leaves or turmeric powder
- 15 drops or evening primrose oil, carrot seed oil, or neem oil
- 1 tsp olive or coconut oil (optional but moisturizing)

Add aloe vera juice, carrot juice, water or chamomile tea to this mix until it forms a dry-ish paste.

Gently apply on circular motions to your skin. Rub on for a few minutes then wash off.

This is a gentle but effective cleanser for your skin.

Skin Balancing Toners

You can rinse your skin now with warm chamomile tea, aloe vera juice (with a few drops of apple cider vinegar added) or baking soda followed by milk and then rinsed with water.

These rinses tone down any PH imbalances and help to soothe and calm skin.

If you want to make an antibacterial wash, use a few drops of tea tree and lavender oil in your rinse with (and this is important) a tsp of apple cider vinegar to balance ph. Adding these oils to either water, aloe vera juice or chamomile tea for a refreshing spritz. Better still soak some rolled oats in the liquid, then strain out the oats leaving the milky liquid.

This is a very soothing recipe that is also great for itchy bites and other itchy skin conditions.

Honey Baking Soda Wash For Removing Makeup

This recipe is one I read about online. It's an excellent recipe but you MUST follow this with an apple cider vinegar toner (1 tsp apple cider vinegar, 1 cup water and a drop or two of lavender essential oil) to rebalance skin afterwards as baking soda will mess with your skins ph.

- 1 tsp baking soda
- 4 Tbsp honey
- 1 cup water

Mix together well and apply with a warm facecloth or cotton ball to your skin. Leave on for a few minutes then wash off and apply the aforementioned apple cider vinegar toner.

Soaps

Just a wee note on soaps, most soaps are drying on skin. Castile soaps on the other hand are vegetable based and gentler on skin but should still be used with care. Glycerin based soaps are preferable if you are going to use them on your body or face as they can be astringent (they close pores and dry out skin).

TONERS

Toners are a lotion or wash for the purpose of cleansing and balancing the skin shrinking the appearance of pores.

Tonic toners are great for acneic skin that may also have issues with dryness. You'll use part astringent and part healing water like rosewater or lavender water or part aloe vera gel. They make your skin feel very clean and help tighten your pores a little. If your skin dries out while using a pure astringent, try turning it into a tonic by diluting it with a healing water.

Toners are usually applied by:

- Dabbing on with cotton wool

- Spraying or spritzing onto the face

- Splashing on to skin

- By applying a gauze facial mask soaked in the toning lotion and left on the face for a few minutes.

Moisturizer is usually followed after toning.

Types of toners

Fresheners and Spritzes

These are the mildest form of toners which normally contain water, hydrosol or a tincture and a humectant such as glycerine. Humectants help to keep the moisture in the upper layers of the epidermis by preventing it from evaporating. Toner hydrosols like Rosewater make excellent toners.

These toners are the gentlest to the skin, and are most suitable for use on dry, dehydrated, sensitive and normal skins. It may give a burning sensation to sensitive skin.

Skin Tonic Toners

These usually contain a small amount of alcohol (up to 20%), water and a humectant ingredient. Orange flower water is one example of this type of toner which is commonly used for normal, combination, and oily skin.

Apply toners by spritzing with a spray bottle or with a cotton pad & leave to dry before applying moisturizer. Can also be used to steam your skin by adding to a steam vaporizer.

Sensitive Skin: Chamomile tea and/or a drop of chamomile oil in a cup of water or tea.

Acneic Skin: 2 drops lavender oil, 2 drops rosemary oil, 1 drop tea tree oil in a cup of water.

Normal or Dry Skin: 2 drops rose oil, 1 drop sandalwood oil, 1 drop palma rosa oil (optional) in a cup of water.

Normal or Oily Skin: 2 drops orange oil (or lemon), 1 drop neroli oil, 2 drops chamomile oil or use 1 cup of chamomile tea instead of a cup of water for the whole recipe.

Astringent Toners

These are the strongest type of toner and may contain a high proportion of alcohol (20-60%). They also can contain antiseptic ingredients, essential oils, fruit extracts/acids, water, and a humectant ingredient.

These are most often recommended for oily skins as they can be drying, removing excess oil from the skin which can lead to excess oil production as the skin tries to compensate for the loss of moisture in the skin.

Witch hazel is an astringent. To prevent dehydration, astringent is best applied only to problem areas of skin, such as pimples and acne.

Natural Toner Examples Include

Witch hazel

Aloe vera

Apple cider vinegar

Hydrosols (left over bi product of essential oil distillation)

Orange oil (acne and oily skin)

Fennel oil (anti-aging)

Rose oil (very hydrating for dry skins)

Frankincense oil (anti aging and firming)

A few drops of the following oils above can be added to water as a toner depending on what skin type you have.

Aloe vera juice or gel

Apple cider vinegar

Black tea

Chamomile tea

Green tea (nice and mild)

Lemon juice

Strawberries

Tomato juice

Vodka (don't use the cheap stuff) when diluted with water is a great toner but can dry out your skin so use carefully

Witch hazel

Witch hazel and apple cider vinegar ½ and ½ as a toner

Hydrosols (Flower Waters) As Toners

Hydrosols are a product of essential oil distillation process

Benefits: Spray spritzing bottles, toners and for hydration. Can be added to moisturizers and toners.

Benefits for skin: They are generally very gentle and soft for your skin

There are many hydrosols listed below:

Chamomile: Soothing calming floral type fragrance, good for sensitive irritated weathered or mature skins.

Clary sage: Perfect for dry and aging skin, clary sage relieves skin problems associated with hormone issues and menopause.

Rose: Balancing astringent properties, again good for sensitive irritated or environmentally damaged skin.

Lavender: An astringent, calming and has antiseptic qualities so its good for acneic or irritated skin and wind or sunburnt skin.

Neroli: Freshly fragranced (orange blossoms) good for sensitive irritated or environmentally damaged skin as well as acneic or irritated and wind or sunburnt skin.

Cucumber Aloe Toner

This is a calming soothing toner that has mild drying qualities.

Juice from half a medium sized cucumber mixed with 2 Tbsp aloe vera juice or gel

Sieve out the cucumber pulp and mix the juices together. Apply with a cotton ball or by splashing on your skin and allowing to dry.

Easy Lavender Toner

Moisturizing and soothing – the easiest toner ever

- 2 cups witch hazel
- 6 drops lavender essential oil
- sprig of fresh rosemary or basil of you have it handy

Mix well and store in a spray bottle in the refrigerator. Spray on hair and skin for a refreshing moisturizing boost.

 Keeps up to 5 weeks.

Green Lemon Zest Tea Toner

This can cause photosensitivity so use sparingly in summer

3 Tbsp lemon juice

2 cups strong green tea with lemon (or add a little lemon zest)

3 drops tea tree essential oil (optional) or lavender oil

Combine well by shaking and store in the fridge. Use by spraying or dabbing on skin and allowing to dry before applying moisturizer. Avoid the sun for an hour or two after using this recipe.

Acne Face Toner Recipe

Benefits: Antiseptic, Antifungal, Antibacterial, Balancing, Toning

- 4oz Witch Hazel
- 10 drops tea tree oil

Mix ingredients well in bottle. Shake before each use and apply to skin with cotton ball after cleansing.

FACIAL STEAMS

Steams open pores allowing deep cleansing to remove impurities. The steam process also aids deep penetration of beneficial nutrients into your skin.

Be cautious when using steams on open sores and weeping spots as this process can aggravate them. Wait a day for the lesion to seal over first.

- For a purifying steam add a tsp of salt (rock salt or dead sea salt is great for this) to your water. This is antibacterial and also clears pores.
- For a soothing recipe add a Tbsp of honey.
- For a potent acne recipe, add 4 drops of eucalyptus and tea tree oil (the eucalyptus can be a bit rough on your eyes so only add a drop or two of this).

How To Use Steams

Use a pot of steaming/simmering water or a vaporizer. If using a pot use a large flat one with small handles on each side or if using a pot with one handle, turn it to the back away from you. This is so that you do not accidentally catch a towel or any other accessories that you will be using on the edge of the handle and topple the pot. Simmer on low heat and remove or turn off just before using your steam.

If you do not want to steam your face, use the liquid on a face cloth, and allow to cool enough to apply to your face.

STEAM RECIPES

Oily Skin Steam

- Peel of one lemon
- Few drops of lavender oil (or use fresh lavender stalks)
- Sprig of fresh rosemary

Add these ingredients to a pot of boiling water. Simmer for ten minutes then turn down. Place your face over the steam (very carefully) with a towel draped over your head. Steam for ten minutes.

If using a vaporizer, add the strained liquid to the machine and use as directed.

Chamomile Peppermint Steam

This recipe is good for inflamed skin and also great for headaches.

- 2 cups chamomile tea
- 3 drops peppermint oil

Add these ingredients to a pot of boiling water. Simmer for ten minutes then turn down. Place your face over the steam (very carefully) with a towel draped over your head. Steam for ten minutes.

If using a vaporizer, add the strained liquid to the machine and use as directed.

Coffee Honey Cabbage Steam

- 1 cabbage leaf
- 1 tsp honey

- 3 Tbsp ground coffee (antioxidants and clarifying)

Add these ingredients to a pot of boiling water. Simmer for ten minutes then turn down. Place your face over the steam (very carefully) with a towel draped over your head. Steam for ten minutes.

If using a vaporizer, add the strained liquid to the machine and use as directed.

FACIAL MASK RECIPES

Toothpaste And Baking Soda (Or Aspirin)

This an oldie but goodie. Mix equal parts baking soda and toothpaste as a spot treatment. You can also add a few drops of tea tree oil, honey and turmeric powder to boost its potency. You can also use crushed (uncoated) aspirin as an alternative.

Saline Solution

A solution of salt water, with or without vinegar, can help clear up your acne both by drying your skin (removing excess oils) and by helping to disinfect it. Wash your face twice a day with a salt water (and vinegar if you like) solution. Just don't make the remedy too strong, mildly salty is best. For stubborn spots, make a stronger solution, apply to the swollen area, and leave on for 15-20 minutes.

Strawberries And Tomatoes

Strawberries and tomatoes are rich in salicylic acid. Other fruits are high in alpha hydroxyl acids. Both types of acids are great for combatting acne. If you add a few drops of essential oils to a fruit mask made of these fruits, you can enjoy a powerful fruit peel that leaves your skin clean and fresh while fighting acne bacteria.

Add some willow bark powder (see our store for where to find this online) for an extra salicylic acid boost.

Herby Acne Home Remedies

Herbs great for acne include fennel, fenugreek turmeric, garlic and ginger, radish or sesame seeds which can all be added to masks or made into a paste. You can also add these to green or chamomile tea as a steam or toner.

Eat These Herbs As Well

You can also eat the aforementioned herbs in your diet to boost your immune system from the inside out.

Sandalwood Powder

All you need for this remedy is one tsp of sandalwood powder and one tsp of turmeric powder mixed with a Tbsp of honey or yogurt. It forms a paste and is an excellent spot treatment for pimples.

The Oiled Up Strategy

Mix coconut oil and castor oil and olive oil in equal parts with 1% tea tree or lavender oil is a great oil treatment for skin. It is full of antioxidants and antibacterial properties. Plus it's VERY moisturizing for skin.

Acne Apple Cider Vinegar For Pimples

Benefits: Acne, Anti-Oxidant, Cleansing, Exfoliating, Moisturizing, Tightening

Apply straight apple cider vinegar carefully with a Q-tip to each pimple once or twice daily. This helps to quickly dry pimples, prevent spreading, calm inflammation and redness.

Acne Apple Mask

Benefits: Acne, Anti-aging, Age Spots, Anti-oxidant, Anti-fungal, Antiseptic, Antibacterial, Balancing, Cellulite, Calming, Cleansing, Exfoliating, Itchy Skin Moisturizing, Soothing, Tightening

- 2 Tbsp mashed apple or pear
- 1 tsp crushed rosemary, sage or lavender leaves
- Pinch of salt or baking soda

Mash together well (cooked or raw is fine) then apply to your skin. Leave on for 10 minutes then rinse off.

Acne Apple Soothing Mask

Benefits: Acne, Age Spots, Anti-fungal, Anti-oxidant, Balancing, Brightening, Cleansing, Cooling, Dark Circles, Discoloration, Exfoliating, Itchy Skin, Lightening, Moisturizing, Puffiness, Soothing, Tightening

- ½ Cup oatmeal finely ground
- ½ A ripe apple
- 3 Tbsp crushed cucumber
- 2 Tbsp milk

Mix the ingredients together in a blender and apply to skin. Leave on for 20 minutes then wash off with warm water.

Acne Aspirin Mask

Benefits: Anti-aging, Anti-inflammatory, Anti-oxidant, Balancing, Calming, Cleansing, Exfoliating, Healing, Mature Skin, Moisturizing, Repairing, Scarring

- 1-3 aspirin
- 1/3 cup warmed honey
- 3 Tbsp almond, olive or coconut oil

Crush aspirin and add to oil and honey. Apply to skin and leave on for 10-15 minutes then rinse off.

Acne Baking Soda And Toothpaste Spot Cream

Benefits: Age Spots, Anti-Aging, Anti-Inflammatory, Discoloration, Itchy Skin

- 1 tsp of baking soda
- 2 Tbsp water
- ½ tsp toothpaste

Mix ingredients together to form a paste and dab on spots. Clears up pimples quickly.

Acne Basil Blemish Treatment

Benefits: Acne, Anti-Oxidant, Cleansing

- 1 cup water
- ¼ C basil
- 1 Tbsp crushed mint leaves

- ¼ Watercress crushed
- 3 medium size carrots (peeled and chopped)
- 1 egg white

Simmer all ingredients except egg white for 20 minutes on low heat. Remove from heat and allow to cool. Blend all ingredients with the egg white on medium speed for 45 seconds.

Apply to face. Let sit for 10 to 20 minutes. Rinse off with warm water.

Acne Clay Mask

Benefits: Acne Anti-aging, Anti-fungal, Anti-inflammatory, Anti-oxidant, Brightening, Calming, Cleansing, Exfoliating, Healing, Lightening, Mature Skin, Moisturizing, Repairing, Scarring, Soothing

- 3 tsp green clay (if skin is sensitive, use french green clay)
- 1 tsp honey
- 2 Tbsp water (oily skin), half and half (combination skin) or jojoba oil (dry skin)

As a general rule use 2 parts liquid to 1 part clay.

Use the liquid to suit based on your skin type. If you have oily skin use water. Combination skin milk or half and half and for dry skin use jojoba oil.

Mix the ingredients together and apply to skin. Leave on for 10-20 minutes then rinse off with luke warm water.

Acne Eau De Cologne And Lemon Juice

Mix equal quantities of eau de cologne and lemon juice. Apply this solution on the pimples with a Q-tip and leave it to dry reapplying a new layer every five minutes. Wash off after 15-20 minutes.

Acne Egg White And Lemon Mask

Benefits: Anti-oxidant, Anti-aging, Cleansing, Discoloration, Exfoliating, Lightening, Oily Skin, Tightening

- 1 egg white
- 4 drops of lemon juice or essential oil

Separate the egg white from the yolk. Beat the egg white until it forms into soft peaks. Apply to skin and rinse off with warm water.

Acne Fruit Herbal Mask

Benefits: Anti-fungal, Anti-aging, Anti-oxidant, Anti-inflammatory, Antiseptic, Brightening, Cleansing, Discoloration, Exfoliating, Insect Repellant, Lightening, Mature Skin, Moisturizing, Soothing, Soothing, Tightening, Wrinkles

- 1 tsp lemon, orange, or grapefruit juice
- Couple of crushed basil leaves
- 1 Tbsp cream, yoghurt, milk
- 1 avocado
- 1 Tbsp ground almond meal

Blend together to a fine mash with a blender or mortar and pestle. Apply to skin and leave on for 10 to 15 minutes then rinse off.

*Optional extras: 2 drops tea tree oil, manuka oil, rosemary oil or lavender oil

*Alternative base: use mashed apple, papaya, or pineapple.

Acne Green Clay Mask

Benefits: Anti-aging, Balancing, Cleansing, Healing, Itchy Skin,

Moisturizing, Scarring, Wrinkles

- 1 Tbsp green clay from any health store
- 1 tsp apricot kernel oil
- 3 drops of palma rosa essential oil

Mix the ingredients together and apply to skin. Leave on for 10-20 minutes then rinse off with luke warm water.

Acne Honey And Yoghurt Moisturizing Acne Mask

Benefits: Anti-aging, Anti-fungal, Anti-inflammatory, Anti-oxidant, Calming, Cleansing, Exfoliating, Healing, Mature Skin, Moisturizing, Repairing, Scarring, Soothing

- 1 tsp of warmed honey
- 1 tsp of plain yoghurt

Mix the ingredients together and apply to skin. Leave on for 10-20 minutes then rinse off with luke warm water.

Acne Honey Pimple Remedy (Healing And Moisturizing)

Benefits: Anti-aging, Anti-inflammatory, Anti-oxidant, Calming, Cleansing, Exfoliating, Healing, Scarring, Mature Skin, Moisturizing, Repairing

- 3 Tbsp honey
- 1 tsp cinnamon

Mix the ingredients together and apply to infected areas or spots. Can be washed off after 20 minutes if you wish.

Acne Juice Mask

Benefits: Anti-aging, Anti-inflammatory, Anti-oxidant, Blackheads, Brightening, Calming, Cleansing, Exfoliating, Healing, Lightening, Mature Skin, Moisturizing, Oily Skin, Repairing, Scarring, Tightening, Wrinkles

- 1 tsp lemon juice
- 2 egg whites
- 3 tsp honey
- 1 cup strawberries

Mash & mix the ingredients together and apply to skin. Leave on for 10 minutes then rinse off with luke warm water.

Acne Milk Of Magnesia

Benefits: Acne, Anti-fungal, Exfoliating, Lightening, Brightening, Moisturizing, Soothing

1 bottle Milk of Magnesia applied with a cotton ball or pad. Leave on for 10-20 minutes and rinse off.

Acne Milk Soothing Mask

Benefits: Acne, Anti-aging, Anti-fungal, Anti-inflammatory, Anti-oxidant, Balancing, Brightening, Calming, Cleansing, Cooling, Exfoliating, Healing, Lightening, Mature Skin, Moisturizing, Repairing, Scarring, Soothing

- 1 tsp powdered milk
- 1 Tbsp runny honey
- 1 tsp aloe vera
- 2 drops essential oil of your choice

Mix the ingredients together and apply to skin. Leave on for 10-20 minutes then rinse off with luke warm water.

Acne Nutmeg Pimple Remedy

Benefits: Acne, Anti-fungal, Brightening, Exfoliating, Lightening, Moisturizing, Soothing

- 1 Tbsp ground nutmeg
- 1 Tbsp milk

Mix the ingredients together and apply to infected areas or spots. Can be washed off after 20 minutes if you wish.

Acne Oatmeal Mask

Benefits: Anti-aging, Anti-inflammatory, Balancing, Cellulite, Cleansing, Itchy Skin, Mature Skin, Moisturizing, Soothing

- 5 five drops of almond oil
- Juice of half a lemon
- 1 egg white
- 1 Tbsp oatmeal powder (ground oatmeal)

Mix all the ingredients in a bowl to make a smooth paste. Add water if it is very thick. Apply it on the face and leave on for 151"20 minutes. Rinse off with luke warm water.

Acne Oil Blend

Benefits: Acne, Anti-aging, Anti-fungal, Anti-inflammatory, Antibacterial, Antiseptic, Balancing, Calming, Cellulite, Cleansing, Healing, Itchy Skin, Mature Skin, Moisturizing, Repairing, Scarring

2 Tbsp jojoba oil or coconut oil (or use grapeseed or any other oil

mentioned in this book as a base oil)

6 Drops Lavender Oil

5 drops tea tree (melaleuca) or manuka oil

1 drop geranium oil (optional)

Blend ingredients together gently and apply to problem areas of the skin or add to a mask. Store in a glass container.

Acne Patchouli Herbal Cleanser

Benefits: Anti-oxidant, Exfoliating, Healing, Moisturizing, Renewing, Rejuvenating, Repairing

- 2 Tbsp ground hazelnuts or 1 Tbsp hazelnut oil
- 2 Tbsp grapeseed oil
- 5 drops myrrh essential oil
- 5 drops patchouli
- 5 drops tea tree oil

Mix ingredients well in bottle. Shake before each use then apply to skin in a circular motion for a minute or two. Rinse off with warm water.

Acne Slippery Elm Mask

Benefits: Acne, Moisturizing, Oily Skin

- 1 oz slippery elm powder
- 3 oz water
- 3 drops tea tree oil (optional) can also use crushed rosemary leaves

Mix ingredients together and apply to skin. Leave on for 10 mins then wash off with warm water.

Acne Strawberry Cleanser

Benefits: Acne, Anti-fungal, Brightening, Exfoliating, Lightening, Moisturizing, Soothing

- 2 Tbsp strawberry yoghurt or
- 1 strawberry and 1 Tbsp plain yoghurt

Mix the ingredients together and apply to skin in a circular motion for 2 minutes. Rinse off with luke warm water.

Acne Strawberry Mask

Benefits: Anti-aging, Anti-inflammatory, Insect Repellant, Discoloration, Moisturizing

- ¼ Cup strawberries
- ¼ Cup sour cream or plain yogurt

Mash the strawberries and yogurt or sour cream together. Apply to face and wash off after 10-15 minutes.

Acne Tea Tree Oil For Pimples

Benefits: Anti-fungal, Antiseptic, Antibacterial, Balancing,, Calming Cellulite, Cleansing, Soothing

- 15 drops tea tree oil
- 5 drops lavender oil
- 5 drops water

Blend ingredients together. Apply to each pimple a few times a day with a q-tip to quickly dry out pimples.

Acne Tomato Face Mask

Benefits: Acne, Anti-fungal, Balancing, Brightening, Cooling, Calming, Dark Circles, Discoloration, Exfoliating, Itchy Skin, Lightening, Moisturizing, Puffiness, Oily Skin, Repairing, Tightening, Moisturizing

- 1 mashed tomato with seeds removed
- 2 tsp plain yoghurt
- 1 tsp mashed cucumber
- 1 tsp aloe vera gel
- 2 tsp oatmeal
- 2 crushed mint leaves

Mix the ingredients together and apply to skin. Leave on for 10 minutes and wash off. Also great for oily skin.

Acne Turmeric And Honey Mask

Benefits: Acne, Anti-aging, Anti-fungal, Anti-inflammatory, Anti-oxidant, Brightening, Calming, Cleansing, Exfoliating, Healing, Lightening, Mature Skin, Moisturizing, Repairing, Scarring, Soothing

- 1 tsp of natural (not powdered) milk
- 1 tsp of honey
- 1 tsp of turmeric

Mix the ingredients together and apply to skin. Leave on for 10-20 minutes then rinse off with luke warm water.

Acne Rejuvenating Repairing Seaweed Mask

Benefits: Acne, Balancing, Blackheads, Calming, Cooling, Moisturizing, Repairing

- 4 Tbsp kelp powder
- ½ Cup of aloe vera gel or juice
- 3 Tbsp distilled water

Combine dry ingredients adding water gradually until the mixture has a consistency of a thick paste.

Apply on the face and neck and leave it on for about 15 minutes. Rinse off with warm water.

Acne Calming Oily Skin Mask

Benefits: Acne, Balancing, Cooling, Calming, Moisturizing, Repairing

- ½ Cup aloe vera gel
- 1 ½ Tbsp cornstarch
- 1 Tbsp witch hazel
- 3-4 drops peppermint oil

Mix aloe, cornstarch and witch hazel in glass bowl. Microwave in 3 to 4 30 second intervals stirring every interval or cook in a double boiler stirring constantly until it forms a light paste. Store in refrigerator and apply as needed then rinse off with water.

Anti-Fungal Antiseptic Skin Blend

Benefits: Healing, Moisturizing, Soothing

- 7 drops tea tree oil
- 4 drops lavender oil
- 8 drops neem oil or karanja oil
- 20 drops olive oil or almond, or apricot oil

Blend the oils together and apply to affected areas twice daily with a cotton pad or q-tip.

Anti-Fungal Soothing Skin Remedy

Benefits: Acne, Anti-aging, Anti-fungal, Anti-inflammatory, Antibacterial, Antiseptic, Balancing, Brightening, Calming, Cellulite, Cleansing, Exfoliating, Healing, Insect Repellant, Itchy Skin, Lightening, Mature Skin, Moisturizing, Repairing, Scarring, Soothing

- 2 drops karanja oil or neem oil
- 3 drops lavender oil
- 3 drops tea tree oil or manuka oil
- 2 drops rosemary oil (optional)
- 2 Tbsp milk
- 2 Tbsp olive oil

Mix and soak infected area in this mixture with cotton pads. Wash off with warm water if you prefer. Great for tinea and ringworm.

Anti-Fungal Yoghurt, Rosemary, Honey & Lavender Remedy

Benefits: Acne, Anti-aging Anti-fungal, Antiseptic, Antibacterial, Calming, Healing, Moisturizing, Soothing

- 5 drops lavender oil
- ½ Cup yoghurt
- 1 Tbsp honey
- 5 drops rosemary oil

Mix ingredients together and rub onto affected areas then rinse off after 10 minutes.

Acetylsalicylic acid (the chemical name for aspirin) is an anti-inflammatory. When applied to the skin, it will reduce inflammation and can also relieve pain. If you use powdered aspirin you'll also get the stimulating benefits of caffeine, which is great for skin.

- ½ tsp aspirin powdered or tablets crushed

- ¼ tsp of water
- ½ tsp of oil (olive, almond, safflower of any other oil mentioned in this book will do)
- ½ tsp of honey

Mix the ingredients together and apply to skin. Leave on for 10-20 minutes then rinse off with luke warm water.

Anti-Inflammatory Oil Blend

Benefits: Anti-Septic, Anti-Bacterial, Anti-Inflammatory, Moisturizer

- 10 drops rosehip oil
- 5 drops calophyllum oil
- 3 drops myrhh oil
- 10 drops almond oil

Blend oils together and rub in to affected areas as needed. Store in glass bottle.

Anti-Inflammatory Peppermint Mud Mask

Benefits: Anti-Aging, Anti-Inflammatory, Discoloration, Insect Repellant

- 2 Tbsp rubbing alcohol or vodka
- 1 tsp peppermint extract
- 2 tsp fuller's earth (clay)

Mix all ingredients together. Apply to face, avoiding eye area. Leave on for 10 minutes. Rinse off with warm water.

Arrowroot Face Mask

Benefits: Acne, Anti-aging, Anti-inflammatory, Anti-oxidant, Brightening,

Calming, Cleansing, Exfoliating, Healing, Lightening, Mature Skin, Moisturizing, Repairing, Scarring, Soothing

- 1 oz fuller's earth
- 2 tsp arrowroot
- 1 tsp finely ground cornmeal
- 1 tsp finely ground almond meal
- Enough honey, apple cider vinegar, or yogurt to form a soft paste.

Mix ingredients together, apply to skin and leave on for 10-15 minutes. Rinse with lukewarm water.

Basic Clay Mask Base (For Adding Other Active Ingredients & Oils To)

Benefits: Blackheads, Oily Skin, Moisturizing

- 2 oz green clay
- 3 tsp cornstarch

Mix ingredients together this base and store in a jar ready for adding oils and other ingredients to. This is a good moisturizing clarifying base.

Bergamot Cold Cream

Benefits: Acne, Anti-aging, Anti-fungal, Anti-inflammatory, Antibacterial, Antiseptic, Balancing, Calming, Cellulite, Cleansing, Cleansing and Lavender, Cleansing essential oil and Lavender, Discoloration, Insect Repellant, Mature Skin, Moisturizing, Soothing

- ½ tsp borax powder
- 1 Tbsp hot distilled water
- ½ Cup almond oil
- 1 Tbsp grated beeswax
- 1 Tbsp rose flower water
- 2 drops bergamot oil

- 2 drops lavender oil

Mix borax powder and distilled water together for about half a minute. Add the almond oil and grated beeswax to a separate heatproof container and heat in a double boiler or microwave for two to three minutes on high so the beeswax is melted. Add rose flower water, bergamot & lavender oils to the borax solution. Stir. Mix all of the ingredients together and blend for a couple of minutes until well combined and consistent in color. Cool and store in glass of plastic containers. Apply as needed.

Scarring Reduction Scar Removing Facial Oil

Benefits: Anti-fungal, Anti-inflammatory, Antibacterial, Antiseptic, Balancing, Calming, Cellulite, Cleansing, Healing, Repairing, Scarring, Soothing

- 1 oz calophyllum (tamanu) oil
- 15 drops galbunam oil
- 15 drops lavender oil

Blend oils together. Apply a little of this oil to your scars with a cotton ball or q-tip after washing your face. When skin has absorbed all the oil you can apply moisturizers or makeup. Used daily this will reduce the appearance of scars: newer scars will heal faster.

Soothing Acne Red Wine Face Mask

Benefits: Anti-fungal, Anti-inflammatory, Antibacterial, Balancing, Calming, Soothing

- 2 Tbsp red wine
- ½ Tbsp aloe vera gel
- 1 Tbsp honey

- 1 Tbsp kelp powder seaweed powder

Mix the Honey and other ingredients together then leave it to rest for 10 minutes so the kelp powder can absorb the wet ingredients. Apply to face and leave on for around 10 minutes then wash off with warm water.

Calming, Clearing Oatmeal Mask

Benefits: Calming , Soothing, Healing

This is very calming soothing mask for inflamed acne flare ups.

- 3 Tbsp finely ground oats
- 2 tsp honey (use UMF honey if you can)
- 2 Tbsp whole (full fat) milk
- 1 tsp yogurt (plain greek) (optional)
- Few drops of essential oil (optional)

Mash into a thick paste and apply to skin for ten minutes then wash off.

Semi-Natural Aspirin-Honey Face Mask

Benefits: Acne, Oily Skin

Aspirin is rich in salicylic acid. This is a quick and easy oily skin acne mask.

- 6 uncoated 100% aspirin tablets
- 2 Tbsp apple cider vinegar
- 2 tsp honey

Mash together well and allow to sit for 3 to 4 minutes. Apply to skin, leave on for ten minutes then wash off.

Toning Oil Reduction Mask

Benefits: Acne, Oily Skin, Firming, Tightening

- 1 egg white
- 1 tsp lemon juice

Whisk egg whites well then add lemon juice. Apply this mask with a cotton ball while lying down with your face facing the ceiling. Leave it on for ten to 15 minutes then wash off with warm water and pat dry.

Parsley Almond Healing Treatment

Benefits: Acne, Anti-microbial, Antibacterial, Calming, Soothing, Healing, Moisturizing

- 3 Tbsp finely ground raw almonds (or prepackaged almond meal)
- Large handful of fresh chopped parsley
- Enough jojoba oil to make a thick paste
- 1 tsp aloe vera gel or juice (optional)

Mix well in a blender. Apply to skin and leave on for 15 minutes then wash off with warm water.

Carroty Yogurt Pimple Mask

Benefits: Acne, Antioxidant, Calming, Exfoliating, Lightening, Healing, Moisturizing, Scar Reduction, Soothing, Stimulating

The vitamin A from the carrots in this recipe help to target acne and heal potential scarring. Brewer's yeast is simulating and helps circulation.

- 2 cup just cooked carrots (don't overcook)

- A little greek or plain yogurt to make a thick paste
- 1 Tbsp brewer's yeast (optional)

Blend or puree together well and apply to skin in a thick layer. Leave on for 15 to 20 minutes or so until dry then wash off with warm water. Remove thoroughly.

Green Clay Clarifying Mask

Benefits: Acne, Blackheads, Oily Skin, Firming

French green clay is the strongest of all clays. It is known for it's ability to remove impurities in your, minimize pores, tone and clarify skin.

- 1 Tbsp french green clay
- 1 Tbsp strong green tea
- Add a pinch of turmeric, neem oil or powder, tea tree or lavender oils for an antibacterial boost
- 1 tsp honey

Mix well together and apply to skin in a thick layer. Leave on for ten minutes or so until dry then wash off with warm water. Remove thoroughly.

Alternative Clay Mask

- 1 Tbsp bentonite or fullers earth clay or kaolin clay
- 3 drops lavender essential oil
- 2 drops tea tree oil
- 4 drops carrot seed essential oil (optional)
- 1 tsp plain yogurt
- 1 Tbsp cooled strong chamomile tea

Mix well together and apply to skin in a thick layer. Leave on for ten minutes or so until dry then wash off with warm water. Remove thoroughly.

Cocoa Coffee Red Wine Facial Mask

Benefits: Acne, Anti-oxidant, Toning, Oily Skin, Firming

Cocoa powder is an excellent skin softener and healing ingredient. Coffee is a powerful antioxidant and red wine helps to dry out pimples. You can also add oils or herbs to this mix for a strong acne fighting treatment.

- 2 Tbsp red wine
- 2 Tbsp cocoa powder
- 2 Tbsp very strong coffee

Mix thoroughly and apply as a thick paste to skin. You can also add real chocolate to this – melted gently of course for a yummy mask. Wash off after ten minutes on your skin.

MOISTURIZER RECIPES

It's important not to forget moisturizing. I know you might have oily skin, but it is still important to replenish your skin with "good" oils and nutrients that nourish and protect your skin from invading bacteria. They also help to lubricate oil/sebum and avoid congestion or blackheads where acne can form.

There are serums, lotions, moisturizers and balms you can use for this job. Many serums can be modified into moisturizers with the addition of beeswax and glycerin. Beeswax is an emulsifier (allows oils and non oily liquids to be mixed), glycerin is a humectant meaning it attracts moisture.

You will be using many of these types of ingredients in the recipes below.

Here is a quick run down of what different skin care product ingredients do for your skin:

Active Ingredients & What They Do

Here's some of the lingo you've probably heard, seen or read in advertising or on the labels of your beauty products.

Alpha Hydroxy Acids (Aha's)

These are fruit acids naturally derived from fruit extracts. They slough off dead skin cells to reveal younger more youthful looking skin. As we age our skins renewal process slows down and these help to replace that process giving your skin a younger appearance.

Antioxidants

Ingredients that contain vitamin A, C end E, green tea, copper, grapeseed, and kinetin help skin by neutralizing or scavenging free radicals which are molecules that destroy skin cells.

Beta-Hydroxy Acids

These work in a similar way as AHA's but are less potent so therefore less irritating to skin. The most common and well known one is Salicylic acid which is used in acne treatments and dandruff shampoos.

Botanicals

Ingredients from a naturally derived source (usually plants) believed for centuries to have healing or regenerating powers for the skin. Examples are aloe vera, ginko and ginseng.

Coenzyme Q10

This is a nutrient found in every cell of our body known to be a powerful wrinkle buster.

Most commonly used in aromatherapy to scent products but also as complimentary and healing or regenerating active ingredients in skin care products.

Emollients

Found in moisturizers these ingredients help protect the skin by reinforcing the lower moisture barrier deep in the lower epidermis of the skin. Natural emollients include:Apricot Kernel Oil, Avocado Oil, Borage Seed Oil, Evening Primrose Oil, Grape Seed Oil, Hazel Nut Oil, Hemp Seed Oil, Kukui Oil, Macadamia Nut Oil, Mango Kernel Butter, Organic,, Rose Hip Oil, Organic Sesame Seed Oil, Organic Shea Butter, Organic Sunflower Oil, Safflower Oil, Sesame Seed Oil, Shea Butter, Sunflower Oil, Sweet Almond Oil, Tea Tree Oil, Wheat Germ Oil.

Hypoallergenics

Ingredients that are low allergy producing ingredients in products.

Mattifyers

Ingredients that soak up oil like cornstarch and witch hazel.

Humectants

These are compounds that attract moisture from the air to the skin. Examples are hyaluronic acid, honey, glycerin, glucose & propylene glycol.

Liposomes

Delivery agents to help skin absorb ingredients deeper. Oils rich in essential fatty acids do this job.

Retinols

Products high in Vitamin A, for protection against free radicals and some (Retin A and Retinova) dramatically reduce skin damage from the suns rays.

Non-Comedogenics

Ingredients that don't clog pores and encourage blackheads. The ingredients used in this book are all non-comedogenic.

Anti Fungals And Anti Bacterials

Ingredients that combat bacteria and acne related problems. Essential oils like Rosemary, Neem, Tea Tree and others can be added to beauty products to fight bacterial problems.

Hydrosols

Hydrosols are the "left over" by products of making essential oils. Hydrosols in themselves make great toners and have other properties that are very beneficial for skin.

Infusions Or Teas

Infusions are herbs or other parts of plants, fruits, skins and barks or teas. They make great toners with soothing, calming & many other properties that are very beneficial for skin. Often used in skincare or hair care recipes to compliment ingredient blends with invigorating, sweetening & other beneficial scents and aromas.

Single-Ingredient Moisturizers For Oily Skin

All of the oils below are noncomedogenic, meaning they won't clog your pores, and are beneficial for your skin. Most of these oils are light and easily absorbable (except tamanu oil).

You can use these on their own, but I like using combinations of these oils to make the best use of their individual and synergistic beneficial properties.

- Jojoba oil (closely resembles skin's natural oils)
- Tamanu oil (very thick so is best used diluted with other lighter oils)
- Argan oil
- Vegetable glycerin
- Neem oil (antibacterial and antifungal plus healing)
- Grapeseed oil
- Avocado oil (thick like tamanu oil and great for skin)
- Apricot seed oil
- Rosehip oil (very healing and deeply nourishing)
- Olive oil (healing and nourishing)

Acne Herbal Face Lotion

Benefits: Moisturizing, Anti-inflammatory, Antiseptic, Antibacterial, Exfoliating

- 1 oz. beeswax
- 4 oz hazelnuts or 1 Tbsp hazelnut oil
- 15 drops tea tree oil
- 15 drops myrhh

Melt wax and oil together on warm not hot heat (use a double boiler if you have one), when melted blend thoroughly and allow to cool to a luke warm temperature then add essential oils. Allow to cool completely and store in a glass jar.

Nightly Scar Healing Moisturizer For Acne

A very healing nourishing oil that also targets acne.

- 2 Tbsp jojoba oil
- 2 tsp rosehip oil (great for scars)
- 5 drops tea tree oil
- 1 tsp neem or tamanu oil
- 3 drops lavender essential oil
- 2 drops carrot seed oil (optional, also good for healing)

Mix all ingredients in a small, dark glass bottle and shake well. Store out of direct sunlight and use within 6 months. Use a few drops nightly.

Light Moisturizer (Add Your Own Essential Oils)

A nice light moisturizer for soft skin

- 4 cup distilled water
- 3 Tbsp vegetable glycerin
- 5 drops of your favorite essential oil (lavender, neroli, frankincense)
- Mix all ingredients in a small, dark glass bottle and shake well. Store out of direct sunlight and use within 3 months. Use a little daily.

Acne Serum Moisturizer

Benefits: Anti-aging, Anti-fungal, Antiseptic, Antibacterial, Balancing, Calming, Cleansing, Healing, Scarring, Itchy Skin, Moisturizing, Repairing, Soothing, Wrinkles

- 1 oz apricot kernel oil
- 12 drops lavender oil
- 7 drops tea tree oil
- 1 drop geranium oil

Mix all ingredients in a clear plastic or glass bottle shaking well for 2 minutes then apply 1-2 drops after washing.

Healing Herbal Oil

This is an oil you can (and should) leave to sit before using for a couple of weeks. You can also make this into a lotion after this time by melting 2 Tbsp beeswax pellets and a teaspoon of vegetable glycerin to this.

- 1 cup jojoba oil
- 2 cups dried calendula petals
- 3 Tbsp dried rosemary
- 3 drops carrot seed oil
- 3 Tbsp fennel seeds or 4 drops fennel oil

Put the herbs in a bowl and cover with oil. Crush herbs with the oil and place in a glass container with a lid on it for a week or two.

After this infusion has soaked for a fortnight melt the beeswax with a cup of water and then add oils and stir until cooled. This will set over a few hours. Use as desired.

Store out of direct sunlight and use within 6 months.

My Favorite Acne Serum For Oily Skins

This recipe has everything, it's great for acneic skin but has all the other elements your skin needs without leaving it feeling greasy.

- 3 Tbsp jojoba oil
- 2 Tbsp apricot kernel oil
- 1 tsp borage (starflower) oil
- 2 tsp tamanu oil
- 2 drops neroli or rose oil (optional but very good for keeping wrinkles at bay)

- 1 tsp evening primrose oil or rose hip seed oil
- 5 drops each frankincense, rose geranium, and chamomile essential oils
- 3 drops carrot seed oil (optional also great for healing skin)

Mix all ingredients in a small, dark glass bottle and shake well. Store out of direct sunlight and use within a year. Use after cleansing and you only need a little.

Serious Moisturizer Recipe Tutorial

If you like the idea of making more of your own lotions and moisturizers that you can add acne fighting essential oils to, these are some base oils to use (some you can use after your acne has been dealt with).

Base Oils For Moisturizers

Almond Oil – all skin types

Almond oil is light and nourishing for skin. It doesn't leave a heavy residue because it absorbs quickly. It is nice as a moisturizer base or as a moisturizing facial serum. You can add other oils like rosehip, carrot seed, argan, wheatgerm or borage oil to protect against environmental damage and repair damage.

Argan Oil – damaged skin and anti-ageing

Argan oil contains a high concentration of vitamin E and fatty acids, which help other ingredients absorb deep into the skin layers. It is also an antioxidant making it an all around winner as an ingredient in skin care moisturizers and serums.

Rosehip Oil – repairing and anti-ageing

Rosehip oil is another oil that has regeneration properties and does wonders for ageing damage skin or scarring. You can add it to a base oil for a nourishing moisturizing serum or in moisturizer.

Extra-Virgin Olive Oil – anti-bacterial, anti-ageing and moisturizing

Extra-virgin olive oil is highly moisturizing for skin and it also contains antibacterial properties which make it perfect for an acne treatment. Olive oil is yet another wonderful ingredient you can include in home-made facial moisturizer recipes. Just like jojoba oil it closely resembles the skin's own sebum and can be used with or in place of jojoba oil.

It's quite gluggy in its consistency so you'll need to warm it slightly before adding it to any serum or moisturizer.

Apricot Oil – light moisturizing

Apricot oil is very similar to almond oil in its consistency and can be used in place of Almond oil. almond and oil is an excellent massage oil, or for use as a light moisturizer.

Jojoba Oil - nourishing, anti-aging and repairing

Jojoba is another oil that closely matches the skin's own sebum making it able to absorb into the skin readily and an excellent serum or moisturizer base. Used with rosehip oil, argan oil, carrot or borage oil it makes an amazing anti-ageing serum that also great for softening wrinkles. Blending this oil with the others mentioned above makes for a wonderful moisturizing and antiaging cream.

Carrot Seed Oil – repairing nourishing and anti-ageing

Carrot seed oil is rich in vitamin A making it excellent for repairing sun damaged skin. It's also perfect for rejuvenating dry mature skin. Add about three or 4% carrot oil to your home-made facial moisturizer recipe.

Borage Oil – anti aging and anti-inflammatory

Borage oil is a natural anti-inflammatory making it great for people with skin conditions. The capsules you can buy it to take internally can also be used like vitamin E capsules as an overnight facial treatment by simply opening the capsule and applying the oil to clean skin. Add to your homemade facial moisturizer recipe for a soothing boost.

Grape Seed Oil – great for acneic skin or oily skin and blackheads

Is a really good base oil for oily, acne prone skin or complexions with lots of clogged pores. It absorbs well and doesn't leave your skin feeling oily.

Avocado Oil – dry skin and mature skins

Avocado oil is packed full of essential fatty acids and other nutrients that are highly beneficial for dry and mature skins. You don't need a lot of avocado oil in your blend to enjoy the benefits of this oil.

Safflower Oil – good for blocked pores and mature skins

Safflower oil is high in linoleic acid, I've included this oil because you can use it in skin serums for dry mature skin thanks to its high content of essential fatty acids. More importantly include safflower oil in your diet in the form of salad dressings and other recipes because it has lots of benefits for skin when taken internally.

Soybean Oil – dark circles and puffiness

This oil is perfect as a 1/3 blend in homemade facial moisturizer recipes if you have dark circles around your eyes

So there you have it, my list of favorite oils to use and home-made facial moisturizer recipes. By using these oils and adding a few essential oil ingredients (more on those in a moment) you'll be giving your skin the nourishment and moisturizing effects of top of the line commercial skincare products without having to pay the exorbitant prices for the privilege of using them.

Not only will your skin feel amazing, that you have the peace of mind knowing that you are only using pure and natural ingredients with no potential side-effects.

Making Your Moisturizer

Step 1. Make a simple (3 ingredient) serum that you can use on it's own OR "convert" into homemade facial moisturizer recipes.

Tip: Make sure you only use serums or home-made facial moisturizers on fresh clean skin. Your moisturizers will add not only absorb better, that won't be locking in all of the dirt and oil that's been sitting on your skin from the day before.

Storing your base oils and glass bottles is the best way to keep them fresh and uncontaminated. It's also easier to keep them on hand for when you're ready to make your moisturizer. Some people are content just to use serums as moisturizers but many people are so accustomed to using lotion on the skin that they prefer to use their recipe in that form.

You can buy glass bottles in many shapes and sizes from Mountain Rose Herbs or Sunburst Bottle

Ingredient Number One – The "Base" or "Carrier" Oil

Beeswax – you will need beeswax to make a moisturizer with your serum available from Amazon

Choosing a base oil for your skin type may take a little thought. If you have oily skin, choose a lighter oil like almond or apricot. For dry or mature skins start with jojoba or argan oil. You can also choose a combination of base oils and play around with the mixture until you find a blend that feels right on your skin.

I generally use one to 3 base oils as a starting point and then add other oils like borage, and carrot seed oils when my skin feels like it needs a little more TLC.

Just remember that your base oil is going to be the main ingredient of your blend, so it pays to make a smaller quantity the first time just to see how you like it.

I know this sounds a little vague for those of you who would like me to be more specific, but the fact is the more you experiment with different oils the more addicted you'll find yourself becoming good idea of perfecting your recipe to suit your unique skin. After all there is only one you, and only you will know what feels the best for you.

Okay okay I hear you saying just give me a basic serum to start with!

So here goes....

My absolute two favorite base oils are argan oil and/or jojoba oil. Why? because they are both easily absorbed into your skin without leaving a sticky residue. They are both very moisturising and have anti-ageing benefits so I like to use a 50-50 blend of these oils to start with.

Based on your skin type here is a mini list of oils to suit general skin types (pick yours below).

Argan Oil (perfect for dry, aging, oily, normal, or acne-prone skin)

Jojoba Oil (excellent for dry, aging, oily, normal, or acne-prone skin)

Apricot Kernel Oil (good any skin type, but especially normal, dry, and aging skin)

Sweet Almond Oil (an all encompassing great facial oil, but can take longer to absorb into skin)

Safflower Oil (good all around oil for acne-prone, normal and dry mature skin)

Grapeseed Oil (excellent for normal, oily, or acne-prone skin)

Avocado Oil (used in smaller amounts for dry and aging skin)

Hemp Seed Oil (a light oil good for all skin types)

Olive Oil (a little heavier but good for all skin types)

Your base oil is going to make up around 2/3 of your finished oil blend.

Don't worry, I will show you how to mix them shortly.

Step 2. Adding "active" ingredient essential oils to your natural face moisturizer recipe.

Most of the ingredients I am going to suggest here won't cost you much but there are others that will make you take a deep breath when you get to the checkout.

Fortunately the more expensive – and very optional I might add – ingredients are extremely concentrated and will last you two to three years when using them regularly. More expensive oils like rose oil (it's like liquid gold as a hydrating moisture bath for your skin) and a $20 bottle of concentrated rose oil will give you the same benefits of having a years worth of hydration spa treatments at your local salon.

So relatively speaking, even though you don't need to buy expensive ingredients, the benefits far outweigh the cost compared to the equivalent price of an expensive bottle of skin cream from your local cosmetics counter.

Find your "nourishing oils"

It's absolutely fine if you want to skip adding the nourishing bonus oils but experience tells me that once you get started you'll probably find yourself becoming addicted to the results and want to try more ingredients as an everyday treat for your skin!

So here are some suggestions for nourishing oils to include in your facial recipes:

Tamanu Oil (amazing for acne-prone problem skin)

Neroli Oil (very antiaging and fabulous for red veins or rosacea as is parsley oil/infused parsley leaves in the oil)

Sea Buckthorn Oil (powerful nourishing oil, excellent for all skin types, but especially mature, aging or dry skin)

Evening Primrose Oil (acne, aging, normal skin, hormone balancing and can be taken internally to reduce acne)

Neem Oil (very antimicrobial and healing, neem oil is tops for acne and oily skin)

Emu Oil (a powerful emollient emu oil is protective and nourishing for dry or aging skin)

Extra Virgin Coconut Oil (warm before use as it melts at low room temperatures – great for itchy dry or acne prone skin)

Rosehip Seed Oil (anti-wrinkle oil – highly regenerating and well known for it's firming and anti-aging abilities – perfect for dry, aging, and normal skin)

Carrot Seed Oil (you only need a tiny amount of this oil, but it's superb for any skin type especially scarred damaged skin and wrinkles)

Borage Oil (ridiculously high in oleic acids making it great for most skin types, but especially oily and acneic skin, can go rancid if left in warm or light conditions)

Now, you might want to add a little bit of "flava" with an essential oil!

Step 3. add "active oils

(STOP: IMPORTANT, if you are making moisturizer add these oils AFTER Step 5.)

Remember! You only need a couple of tiny drops of essential oil to get the benefits you need for your skin. Essential oils are potent (and they last for a ridiculously long time when you use them this way)!

Tea Tree Oil (anti-bacterial, anti-fungal and anti-microbial – amazing for acne prone skin but only use a few drops)

Lavender (acne, oily, or dry skin – lavender is soothing healing, you only need a tiny amount)

Peppermint (like lavender, peppermint is great for oily and acneic skin, It's an astringent, and leaves your skin with a tingle)

Chamomile (best to use chamomile is Roman – healing and soothing, so it's great for ALL skin types. Costly though)

Rose Geranium (a healing general essential oil – this is especially good for dry, sensitive skin, mature aging, and normal skin)

Palmarosa (great for any skin type, but perfect for acne prone clogged skin, in addition to being softening and soothing for aging skin)

Lemongrass (brightening and toning, this is a great oil for normal, oily, or acneic skin)

Rosemary (anti-microbial so great for acne prone oily skin)

Rose Oil (extremely hydrating – can use a few drops in a spray bottle of water for a hydrating spritz, perfect for dry mature and aging skin)

Frankincense Oil (good for mature skin – softening, anti aging and good for wrinkles)

Fennel Oil (skin brightening for dull skin and also clearing blocked pores – lifts tires looking skin)

Sandalwood (great for acneic skin and blotchy skin – normal, oily and dry skin)

Step 4. How to create your recipe:

Now we are getting to the fun part! Mixing your recipe. I am going to start with a serum and then show you how to add beeswax to turn your serum into a natural face moisturizer recipe.

- Fill your bottle to 2/3 full with your base oil.
- Add your "nourishing oils" to about 95% of the total volume. When using extra virgin coconut oil warm and add only up to 20% so it doesn't "set" the blend.
- Now add 4-8 drops of essential oil (5%) NO more. Only add 1 percent peppermint oil if you don't want watery eyes or "onion syndrome". Add UP to 3 drops of tea tree oil and 2 drops of lavender if you are using it. You only need a tiny amount of these oils as they are super potent, so remember – even if they smell faint or you think you need more – don't get heavy handed with the essential oils.
- Place cap on top and shake well.

Keep your facial oil in a cool place out of sunlight. They will last for about 9 months.

Important tip: If you are using borage oil this goes rancid fast so only buy a small amount and add it to each batch sparingly.

Step 5. Making your homemade natural face moisturizer recipe:

Wash your hands and all containers (both mixing and storage) as this recipe does not contain preservatives (adding tea tree and neem oil helps it last longer).

- 1/2 cup of your oil serum blend
- 2 tablespoons cosmetic grade beeswax
- 1 cup of warm water (can add aloe juice into the water or carrot juice for added nourishment made up to the cup full)

Warm your oil blend (excluding essential oils in a double boiler) with beeswax until just melted. Stir together well.

Slowly whip in warm water/water juice mix.

Remove from heat while still stirring until the moisturizer "sets". Add essential oils and stir in gently.

There you have it, your own homemade natural facial moisturizer! Add tea tree, lavender or neem as a basic acne recipe –or any other oil you like.

So How And When Do You Use All Of These Recipes?

Don't worry if you are feeling a little worried about what to use for your skin and when.

You are going to want to try these recipes to see what suits you best, but as a rule you can stay with a simple regimen of:

- Washing/Cleansing (daily)
- Toning (daily)
- Moisturizing (daily)
- Exfoliation (every few days)
- Treatment Mask (once or twice weekly)

You can use rubs (rubbing fruit on your skin) as a quick treatment prior to showering.

You can make a scrub and leave in the shower and use it while washing your body.

You can make small amounts of each recipe, and try them to find your favorites.

Experiment – don't be afraid to test and try these recipes. Start simple and then play with the more complex recipes.

WHERE TO BUY INGREDIENTS/RESOURCES

You can find just about everything you need for recipes at Mountain Rose Herbs or..

Amazon have a huge range of products at great prices.

You can also find all of the books and products we recommend when you visit http://astore.amazon.com/bestp03b-20.

There are many wonderful books on essential oil healing and on making your own skin care recipes at home that I highly recommend.

CONCLUSION

All of the recipes in this book and tips were written to give you a full and complete picture of your acne and a comprehensive range of solutions you can use.

I hope you have enjoyed reading the book and making and using the recipes.

Here's to welcoming back your clear gorgeous healthy skin!

PLEASE TELL US WHAT YOU THINK

I am always keen to hear your opinion so I can make any improvements to the context or clarity of the information I provide. I encourage you to leave a review on Amazon. I appreciate all of your reviews so I can add any suggested improvement to the next edition (if I use your suggestion I will send you a free updated edition or another one of my books – your choice).

Thanks so much for reading ☺

ABOUT THE AUTHOR

Mia Gordon is a natural skin care therapies expert, researcher, author and founder of http://www.naturalskincarerecipes.com.

Since 2004 Mia has used her knowledge and passion to research and develop a large range of highly beneficial natural skin care recipes including natural homemade face masks and homemade skincare products.

Mia shares hundreds of easy homemade face masks, skin care recipes, acne treatments, and anti aging oil blends to protect, nourish and beautify skin.

Discover the joy and fun of creating your own homemade personalized body care products using herbs and other natural ingredients that nourish, repair heal, pamper, cleanse, and protect the skin with all natural non irritating ingredients.

INDEX

www.ingramcontent.com/pod-product-compliance
Lightning Source LLC
Chambersburg PA
CBHW070925290526
45795CB00001B/425